Abstract

If you ever saw the movie *One Flew over the Cuckoo's Nest* with Jack Nicholson, this author lived that nightmare. His Story directly documented by the medical manuscripts from Michigan's Coldwater State Home & Training School, will open your eyes to the abuse, neglect and downright ignorance of a mental institution that caged and incarcerated this three-pound baby boy amidst the horrors of institutionalized slavery in the 1950's and 1960's. Still this young man refused to be labeled and went on to achieve a Bachelor's Degree from Western Michigan University and a Master's Degree from Spring Arbor University. All along he was determined to expose this medical horror and achieve his freedom from the depths of hopelessness. Ultimately the author was able to lead a successful life even after emerging from sewers of filth!

THE UNTOLD YET TRUE REMARKABLE STORY OF A VERY DETERMINED LITTLE BOY NAMED JOHNNIE

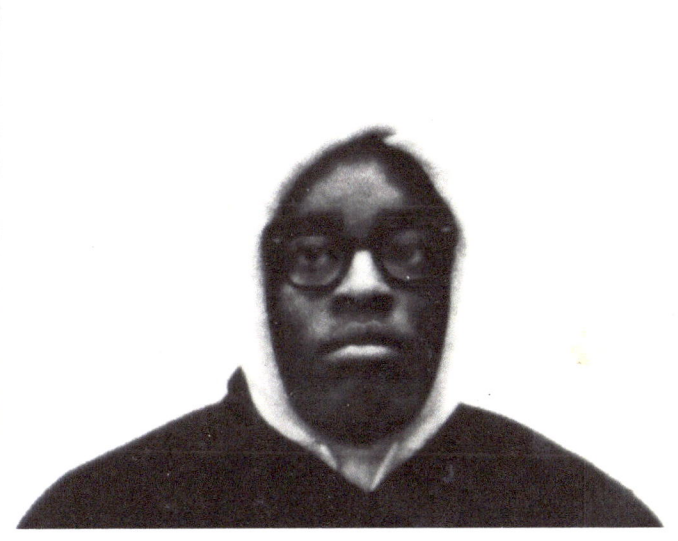

A MEDICAL NIGHTMARE AND HIS MARCH TO FREEDOM

Full Cover Photo by: The Ann Arbor Chronicle: In the Archives: A Coldwater Doll

There is a saying that when someone is discussing you, but they are not in your presence, your ears will burn! If that is so, your ears should have burn many times over the years because I spoke to adults and youngsters about your achievements.

Reading, "The Untold\, Yet Remarkable, Story of a Very Determined little Boy Named Johnnie", I smiled when Bialock in his report mentioned that Sadie Barham was an attractive lady who appeared in her early thirties. She was a very attractive and classy lady. Actually she was forty-four!

I thought there would be a big discussion if Dennis Poole, Terry Schedeler, Curtis Wilson, and if he was still alive, Tony Gillespie had the opportunity to read the comment that you were proud of leading the East Jr. High School basketball team to a 22-0 record!

In the section "Left To Do It Alone" some of my fears were validated when you talked about your life in the Delph's home. I always had a strange feeling about them. Some of the body language and facial expression I saw you , Andy and Charles display may me suspect of just what you described, but I could never get positive proof.

It was depressing to read in the section "My New Home" that you had experienced sexually abuse while at Fort Custer and Allen Elementary School. Was the Teacher at Allen Elementary, Mr. Moore?

Coach John Young

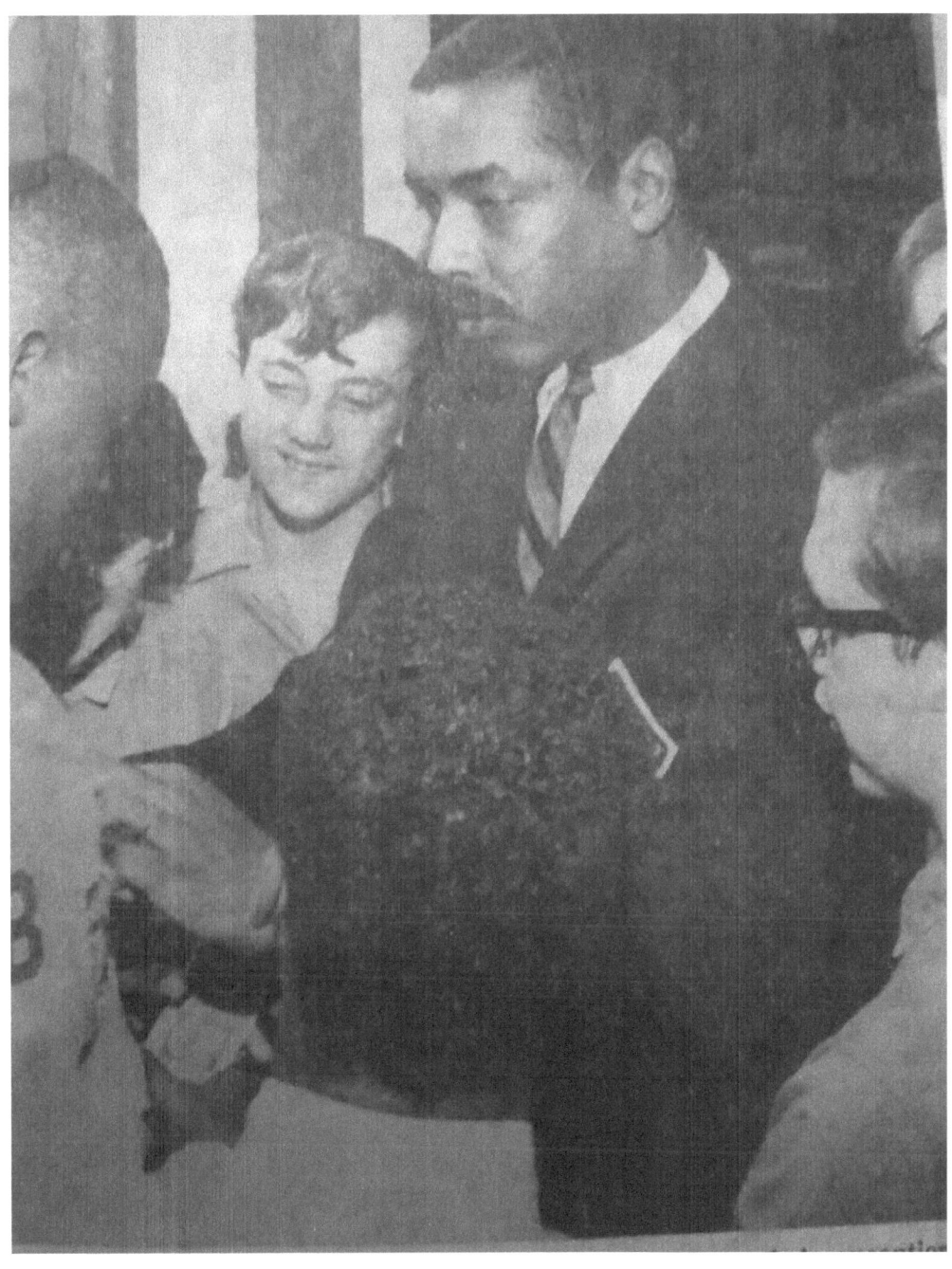

This is Coach John Young, former East Junior High School Special Education Teacher, talking with his 9th grade Special Education Students. That's me with the 1968 varsity letter.

Dear Coach Pharms:

Greetings from your California family, the Archie Moore's & Co. From what my son Hardy has to report about you, you must be quite a swell person. I do believe that God tries his people, knowing full well what their reactions will be.

From the fabulous news releases, you are now on the correct hi-way towards successville, I want to thank you for your interest in my son Hardy, Hardy like I was is a natural athlete, high-strung, and talented, who if he likes someone working hard to to accomplish worthwhile goals, is a dependable player.

A few days ago, Coach Tom Flores sat beside me in the Los Angeles airport and we discussed Hardy's chances to play for the Raiders, I was pleased with what Flores said. So tell my son he is not alone, and all I want form him is to play his part top level at all times.

Coach, you spoke of visiting the Moore's and we welcome you, just lets us know when. Your young lady Julie's from Pittsburg, Kansas, mentioned in your write-up must really special and I often think an honest God- fearing person will eventually reach his goals.

You certainly have put your tome to excellent use, serving the youths. I congratulate you and hope to meet you soon.

In closing, we, the Moore's, with you good speed, adios nos esperanda su tarjeta pronto.

Archie and Mrs. Moore

"OF THE 2,900 PATIENTS AT STATE HOME, SOME 450 ARE BEING TRAINED BY THE SCHOOL IN A VARIETY OF JOBS IN HOPES THAT THEY CAN EVENTUALLY TAKE JOBS AND LEAVE THE INSTITUTION."

"THERE ARE 175 CHILDREN IN THE ACADEMIC PROGRAM. THESE ARE RECEIVING INSTRUCTION FROM TEACHERS WHO ARE CERTIFIED IN THE AREA OF SPECIAL EDUCATION."

(THE COLDWATER DAILY REPORTER. "COLDWATER STATE HOME PLAYS A MAJOR ROLE IN COUNTY ECONOMY," SAT. FEBRUARY 10, 1863, P. 14)

STATE PUBLIC SCHOOL AT COLDWATER

IN 1871, THE MICHIGAN LEGISLATURE AUTHORIZED THE BUILDING OF A SPECIAL STATE PUBLIC SCHOOL TO FURNISH TEMPORARY SUPPORT AND INSTRUCTION FOR DEPENDENT AND NEGLECTED CHILDREN BETWEEN THE AGES OF FOUR (4) AND SIXTEEN (16) UNTIL THY COULD BE PLACED IN HOMES OR RETURNED TO THEIR FAMILIES. THE SCHOOL WAS OPENED IN COLDWATER ON MAY 21, 1874. ONCE ADMITTED, CHILDREN PARTICIPATED IN "FAMILY-LIKE" LIFE IN COTTAGES AND A PLACING-OUT PROGRAM

A THIRD OF EACH DAY WAS USED FOR SCHOOLWORK, A THIRD FOR RECREATION AND ENTERTAINMENT AND A THIRD FOR LEARNING LABOR SKILLS. THEY WERE TAUGHT READING, SPELLING, COUNTING, CALISTHENICS, SINGING, CIPHERING AND SLATE DRAWING. BY THE TURN OF THE CENTURY, THE FACILITY HAD BECOME THE ONLY HOME IN MICHIGAN ADMITTING BOTH NORMAL AND HANDICAPPED CHILDREN.

(MICHIGAN HISTORY DIVISION, DEPARTMENT OF STATE, 1981)

The Untold Yet Remarkable Story of a Very Determined Little Boy Named Johnnie

CASE HISTORY OF JOHN PHARMS #471

ALTHOUGH THE CASE HISTORY INDICATES THAT THE TWINS WERE ONCE MALNOURISHED AND LIVING IN AN IMPROVED EMOTIONAL SETTING, IT NOW APPEARS THAT THE RESILIENCY OF INFANTS HAS ALLOWED THEM MUCH IMPROVEMENT. AT PRESENT, THEY ARE ACTIVE, ALERT, FULL OF QUESTIONS AND ARE TWO OF OUR MOST COLORFUL LITTLE BOYS. DUE TO THEIR ACTIVENESS AND CUTENESS, THEY HAVE BECOME A PAIR OF FAVORITES ON THE WARD, AND THEY LIKE IT.

THEY ARE TOILET TRAINED, FEED THEMSELVES AND PARTIALLY TAKE CARE OF DRESSING THEMSELVES; ALL BUT TYING KNOTS AND ZIPPING ZIPPERS.

BESIDES THE USUAL PATIENT ACTIVITIES, WE HAVE INCLUDED JOHN AND JAMES IN A SPECIAL GROUP. THIS GROUP OF EIGHT TODDLERS THAT ARE LIKELY TO PROFIT FROM AN EDUCATIONAL PROGRAM AT SOME FUTURE DATE, SOME OF WHOM MAY EVENTUALLY BECOME CAPABLE OF INDEPENDENT LIVING. THIS PROGRAM INCLUDES EVERYTHING THAT WE CAN THINK OF THAT IS FUN FOR KIDS. IT IS HOPED THAT THIS WILL STIMULATE PERSONALITY DEVELOPMENT TO THE POINT THAT AN EDUCATIONAL PROGRAM MAY BE AS EFFECTIVE AS POSSIBLE.

INTELLECTUALLY, THE BOYS ARE MEDIUM, RANGE MORONS. JOHN IS SOMEWHAT LARGER THAN JAMES IN PHYSICAL STATURE. BOTH BOYS HAVE EYE DEFECTS, ESPECIALLY JAMES AS HE HELD PICTURES WITHIN FIVE INCHES OF HIS EYES TO SEE THEM. HE WAS RECENTLY SEEN AT THE UNIVERSITY OPHTHALMOLOGY SECTION FOR THIS LAST MENTIONED CONDITION.

In a few years, they both should be given educational opportunities, another evaluation will be indicated at the time.

The type of academic training will depend upon the results of the attempt at the improvement of their vision; either glasses and/or surgery. The fall of 1958, at the earliest, to the fall of 1959 at the latest, seems to be the indicated time period to start their special school training. Present results on the WISC were: Verbal Scale I.Q. = 80; Performance I.Q. = 78, with a Full Scale I.Q. of 77; CA = 7 years 7months, CA – 6 years approximately. A copy of the recent psychological is enclosed.

RECOMMENDATIONS

Since it appears that John is ready for academic training, it is requested that he be transferred to the Coldwater State Home and Training School since we do not have a suitable program for him at Fort Custer.

V. Virginia Young
Director, Social Services

PHARMS, JOHN LEWIS
$471
TRANSFER SUMMARY

ADMISSION

JOHN LEWIS PHARMS WAS COMMITTED BY THE KENT COUNTY PROBATE COURT MAY 1, 1956. HE WAS ADMITTED TO COLDWATER STATE HOME AND TRAINING SCHOOL SEPTEMBER 5, 1956 AND TRANSFERRED TO FORT CUSTER STATE HOME SEPTEMBER 21, 1956. HIS TWIN BROTHER, JAMES LAWRENCE PHARMS, NO.480, IS ALSO A RESIDENT OF THE FORT CUSTER STATE HOME.

FAMILY

THE PARENTS WERE MR. AND MRS. ARTHUR L. PHARMS (GILLIE MAE EZELLE) WHO WERE SEPARATED IN 1953. THE FATHER HAD INTIMATED THAT HE WAS NOT THE NATURAL FATHER AS HE ALLEGES HE WAS IN THE ARMY STATIONED IN ARIZONA AT THE TIME OF CONCEPTION. HE WAS FORMERLY AN EMPLOYEE OF THE KIEFER TANNERY AND WAS HOSPITALIZED AT THE VA HOSPITAL IN ANN ARBOR FROM FEBRUARY 1955 TO JUNE 16, 1956, WHERE HE WAS TREATED FOR TUBERCULOSIS MENINGITIS. AT THE TIME OF HIS SONS' ADMISSION TO COLDWATER, HE WAS UNEMPLOYED AND HIS WHEREABOUTS ARE PRESENTLY UNKNOWN.

THE TWINS WERE REFERRED TO COURT ON A NEGLECT PETITION OCTOBER 31, 1952, AND WERE MADE PERMANENT WARDS OF THE COURT OCTOBER 23, 1953. ON NOVEMBER 6, 1953 THEY WERE PLACED BY THE COURT IN THE CUSTODY AND CARE OF THEIR PATERNAL UNCLE AND AUNT, MR. AND MRS. MATT PHARMS, 22 DELAWARE, GRAND RAPIDS, MICHIGAN. THESE ARE THE ONLY RELATIVES WHO HAVE VISITED THE TWINS IN THE

RESIDENTIAL SETTING AND SINCE THEY WERE GIVEN CUSTODY BY THE COURT, IT WOULD SEEM THAT THEY SHOULD BE CONSIDERED THE NEXT-OF-KIN AND THE PERSON TO BE NOTIFIED IN CASE OF EMERGENCY.

BIRTH AND EARLY DEVELOPMENT

JOHN AND HIS TWIN WERE BORN FEBRUARY 21, 1952 IN GRAND RAPIDS, MICHIGAN, ONE MONTH PREMATURE BY CESAREAN SECTION. BIRTH WEIGHT WAS APPROXIMATELY THREE (3) POUNDS. THE COMMITTING DOCTOR ALLUDED TO THE FACT THAT THE BOYS DID HAVE MENINGITIS BUT NO OTHER INFORMATION IS AVAILABLE REGARDING THIS. AFTER BEING PLACED WITH THE UNCLE AND AUNT, IT WAS APPARENTLY DISCOVERED THAT THE CHILDREN WERE RETARDED AND JOHN'S BEHAVIOR MADE IT NECESSARY TO PETITION FOR COMMITMENT. HE WAS FEARFUL, NERVOUS, NOT OBEDIENT, STUBBORN, FOUGHT WITH THIS TWIN BROTHER, AND WOULD NOT PLAY WITH OTHER CHILDREN.

ADJUSTMENT AT FORT CUSTER STATE HOME

JOHN HAS BEEN GIVEN A DIAGNOSIS OF MENTAL DEFICIENCY; HIGH GRADE MORON; UNDIFFERENTIATED, I.Q. 77. JOHN IS AN ALERT NEGRO BOY IS CONSTANTLY BIDDING FOR ATTENTION. HE IS USUALLY COOPERATIVE AND HELPFUL AND AT TIMES IS VERY DOMINEERING WITH THE OTHER CHILDREN. HE IS ABLE TO CARE FOR HIMSELF. HE AND HIS BROTHER, JAMES, HAVE BEEN INCLUDED IN A PRE-SCHOOL GROUP AS IT WAS ANTICIPATED THAT THEY WOULD EVENTUALLY BE ELIGIBLE FOR AN ACADEMIC PROGRAM. HIS ALTERNATING STRABISMUS DETRACTS ONLY SLIGHTLY FROM HIS APPEARANCE.

MATERNAL SIBLINGS

<u>MOTHER</u>:

GILLIE MAE EZELLE, WAS BORN IN MISSISSIPPI OR TENNESSEE IN 1926. SHE HAS AN EIGHTH (8TH) GRADE EDUCATION. SHE HAS SHOWN LITTLE OR NO CONCERN ABOUT THE CHILDREN. HER PRESENT WHEREABOUTS ARE UNKNOWN. PRIOR TO HER MARRIAGE TO MR. PHARMS, SHE HAD ONE ILLEGITIMATE CHILD. THEY WERE MARRIED JUST TWO MONTHS BEFORE THE BIRTH OF THE FIRST CHILD. SINCE HER SEPARATION FROM MR. PHARMS IN 1953, IT IS ALLEGED THAT SHE HAS LIVED WITH VARIOUS MEN. SHE APPEARS BELOW AVERAGE IN INTELLIGENCE.

THERE IS A HISTORY OF PROMISCUITY AND EVIDENCE OF LOW MORAL STANDARDS IN HER OWN FAMILY.

<u>PATIENT'S SIBLINGS</u>:

1. CHARLES EZELLE, BORN JUNE 18, 1948 IS AN ILLEGITIMATE CHILD OF GILLE MAE. THE ALLEGED FATHER IS WOODLY LESLIE. THE CHILD IS A TEMPORARY WARD OF THE COURT, HE HAD BEEN IN FOSTER CARE SINCE NOVEMBER 1954. ON APRIL 1956, HE WAS RETURNED TO THE CHILDREN'S SHELTER. REFERRAL HAS BEEN MADE TO THE D.A. BLODGETT HOME. PSYCHOLOGICAL REPORTS INDICATE HE HAS AN I.Q. OF 84. HE IS CONSIDERED A BEHAVIOR PROBLEM

The Untold Yet Remarkable Story of a Very Determined Little Boy Named Johnnie

1. ARTHUR LEE PHARMS, BORN OCTOBER 28, 1950, HAD A TWIN SISTER WHO DIED SHORTLY AFTER BIRTH. HE IS ALSO A TEMPORARY WARD OF THE COURT. HE HAS BEEN IN RELATIVES' HOMES AND A LICENSED BOARDING HOME SINCE AUGUST 1955. HE HAS BEEN A DISTURBED CHILD AND WAS REFERRED TO THE CHILD GUIDANCE CLINIC. HE WAS EXAMINED THERE ON MARCH 20, 1956. ON THE STANFORD-BINET, FORM L, ARTHUR EARNED A MENTAL AGE OF 3 YEARS, 10 MONTHS AND AN I.Q. OF 71. HE IS HYPERACTIVE AND VERY DISTRACTIBLE. THE CHILD GUIDANCE CLINIC FELT HE SHOULD HAVE A PSYCHIATRIC EVALUATION.

2. JAMES LAWRENCE PHARMS, TWIN TO THE PATIENT, WAS ADMITTED TO THE COLDWATER STATE HOME AND TRAINING SCHOOL ON THE SAME SATE AS JOHNNY. HIS I.Q. IS 63 AND HIS FILE NUMBER IF [IS] #4422.

3 AND 4

TWINS, NAMES AND SEX NOT LEARNED, WERE BORN ON FEBRUARY 27, 1953. THEY DIED ON MAY 1, 1953, CAUSE UNKNOWN.

PATERNAL SIBLINGS:

1. LILLIAN PHARMS KELLY, COMPLETED SOME HIGH SCHOOL WORK.

2. MILDRED PHARMS THOMPSON, COMPLETED HIGH SCHOOL.

3. DAVID PHARMS, ATTENDED HIGH SCHOOL, BUT DID NOT COMPLETE HIS STUDIES.

4. FRANK PHARMS, COMPLETED HIGH SCHOOL, AND MAY HAVE COMPLETED COLLEGE.

5. MALISIA PHARMS, COMPLETED HIGH SCHOOL.

6. ETHEL L. PHARMS, COMPLETED HIGH SCHOOL.

7. WILLIE MAE PHARMS, COMPLETED HIGH SCHOOL.

8. FRANKIE B. TURNER, COMPLETED HIGH SCHOOL

9. MATT PHARMS, BORN 12/18/31, COMPLETED HIGH SCHOOL. HE SERVED IN THE ARMY FROM JULY 1952 UNTIL THE FALL OF 1954. HE HAS A QUIET PERSONALITY, DOES NOT SMOKE OR DRINK, AND PRESENTLY IS EMPLOYED AS A CONSTRUCTION WORKER. HE AND HIS WIFE, JULIA HALL PHARMS, ACCEPTED THE TWINS IN THEIR HOME WITH THE IDEA THAT EVENTUALLY THEY WOULD ADOPT THEM. THEY HAVE ONE DAUGHTER BORN IN NOVEMBER, 1955.

10. HAROLD PHARMS, BORN IN MARCH, 1934, COMPLETED HIGH SCHOOL

NOTE:

IT IS FELT THAT SOME OF THESE PEOPLE ARE RELATIVES BY MARRIAGE. IT IS KNOWN THAT MATT AND HAROLD ARE HALF SIBLINGS TO THE TWIN'S FATHER.

FATHER:

ARTHUR L. PHARMS WAS BORN NOVEMBER 4, 1921 IN MILLICAN, TEXAS, HE COMPLETED HIGH SCHOOL. HE MARRIED GILLIE MAE EZELLE ON AUGUST 29, 1950 IN GRAND RAPIDS, MICHIGAN, AND WAS SEPARATED FROM HER IN 1953. HE PREVIOUSLY EXPRESSED MUCH CONCERN OVER THE CHILDREN. HE FELT THEIR MOTHER WOULD NEVER GIVE THEM ADEQUATE CARE AND BELIEVED THAT AN ADOPTIVE PLACEMENT FOR THE TWINS WOULD BE DESIRABLE. HE HAS INTIMATED THAT HE WAS NOT THE NATURAL FATHER OF THE TWINS AS HE ALLEGES HE WAS IN THE ARMY STATIONED IN ARIZONA AT THE TIME OF CONCEPTION. IN FEBRUARY 1955, HE BECAME ILL WITH TUBERCULOSIS MENINGITIS AND WAS HOSPITALIZED AT THE VETERAN'S HOSPITAL IN ANN ARBOR. HE PRESENTLY IS UNEMPLOYED, HAVING BEEN DISCHARGE FROM THE HOSPITAL ON JUNE16, 1956. PRIOR TO HIS HOSPITALIZATION, HE WAS EMPLOYED AS A JANITOR AT THE KIEFER TANNERY. HIS EMPLOYER STATED THAT HE WAS

WELL THOUGHT OF, BUT THAT MRS. PHARMS CONTINUALLY RAN HIM INTO DEBT, AND THERE WERE NUMEROUS GARNISHMENTS ON HIS WAGES. IT IS REPORTED THAT HE DRANK EXCESSIVELY ON HIS CONVALESCENT LEAVES FROM THE HOSPITAL.

COLDWATER STATE HOME AND TRAINING SCHOOL

JUNE 1962

MUSIC:

(JOHN'S) SPEECH IS A LITTLE PROBLEM TO HIM, BUT DOES NOT SEEM TO BOTHER HIS COMMUNICATION WITH OTHER STUDENTS.

WORD MASTERY

FAIR BUT INACCURATE AND BOTHERED BY SPEECH IMPEDIMENT. JOHN HAS AN EYE HANDICAP.

PSYCHOLOGICAL REPORT

RETEST

APRIL 9, 1964

ACCORDING TO THE RESULTS OF THIS TEST, JOHN FUNCTIONS INTELLECTUALLY IN THE MENTALLY DEFECTIVE RANGE, AT THE LOW GRADE MORON LEVEL. IT APPEARS THAT HIS VISUAL MEMORY, VISUAL-MOTOR COORDINATION AND CONCEPTUAL ABILITY ARE QUITE LIMITED; WHILE MEMORY FOR MEANINGFUL MATERIAL (AUDITORY MEMORY), WORD FLUENCY AND VOCABULARY ARE RELATIVELY GOOD FOR HIS MENTAL AGE.

The Untold Yet Remarkable Story of a Very Determined Little Boy Named Johnnie

PATIENT'S PROGRESS AT CSH & TS:

PRE-ADMISSION RECORDS INDICATE THAT JOHN AND HIS TWIN WERE VICTIMS OF A VERY DEPRIVED AND UNSTRUCTURED LIVING PATTERN. AFTER BEING TAKEN FROM THEIR PROMISCUOUS MOTHER BECAUSE OF EXTREME PHYSICAL AND EMOTIONAL NEGLECT THEY WERE ADMITTED TO OUR INSTITUTION. IT IS FELT THAT JOHN'S STAY IN THE STRUCTURED INSTITUTIONAL ENVIRONMENT HERE HAS CONTRIBUTED GREATLY TO HIS PROGRESS, AND THAT A FAMILY CARE PLACEMENT IN A STRUCTURED, ACCEPTING HOME SUCH AS THE DELPHS, WILL FURTHER STIMULATE HIM TO REACH HIS FULL POTENTIAL ACADEMICALLY AND SOCIALLY.

MAY 14, 1964:

DISCUSSED BY COMMITTEE COMPOSED OF DR. WISE, DR. WALTON, DR. GEIB, DR. HEINRICH, MR. HARRIS, MRS. BRADLEY AND MISS COX. PLACEMENT IN FAMILY CARE WAS APPROVED. THERE WAS CONSIDERABLE DISCUSSION ABOUT THE SEPARATION OF THE TWINS WITH DR. WALTON ASKING THAT HIS NOTE AGAINST SEPARATION BE MADE A MATTER OF RECORD. THE MAJORITY FELT SEPARATION TO BE NECESSARY AT THIS TIME, BUT THAT VISITS SHOULD BE ARRANGED WITH FAIR FREQUENCY, UNDER THE PLAN AS OUTLINED BY SOCIAL SERVICES.

PSYCHOLOGICAL REPORT

DATE OF TESTING: 8-25-58

RE-EXAMINATION:

JOHN WAS RE-TESTED THIS MORNING AND JAMES THIS AFTERNOON. WITHIN THE LAST YEAR IT HAS BECOME MORE APPARENT THAT JOHN IS PACING HIMSELF AHEAD OF HIS TWIN BROTHER IN TERMS OF MATURITY AND MENTALITY.

IN THEIR DAILY ACTIVITIES, JOHN WATCHES OVER JAMES TO A NOTICEABLE DEGREE, BEING CAREFUL TO SEE THAT JAMES GETS HIS CLOTHES ON CORRECTLY, GETS TO THE MOVIES AND TO MEALS ON TIME, ETC. WHEREAS JOHN GETS GROUPS STARTED WITH GAMES, JAMES WILL STAY AT AN ACTIVITY FOR JUST A VERY FEW MINUTES.

IN THE TEST SITUATION, JOHN WAS JUST A LITTLE OVER ACTIVE AS HE LOOKED ABOUT THE OFFICE FOR THINGS TO LOOK AT AND TO ASK QUESTIONS ABOUT. YET HE SEEMED CONFIDENT ABOUT WHAT HE WAS DOING. WHEN ASKED TO DRAW A PICTURE OF A PERSON, HE PRODUCED ONLY PARTIALLY ORGANIZED CIRCLES AND LINES BUT MADE ELABORATE VERBAL COMMENTS AS HE PROCEEDED, SUCH AS "THIS IS HIS SHOES, SOCKS, GET FIXED UP IN GOOD CLOTHES," ETC. AS HE FINISHED, HE APPEARED PLEASED WITH HIS SPOTTY FIGURE, INDICATING A RETARDED PERCEPTUAL APPRECIATION.

QUALITATIVELY, HIS FIGURE OF A PERSON WOULD BE AVERAGE FOR A FOUR YEAR OLD SHOWING A VISUAL PERSPECTIVE LAG, HOWEVER, ON THE VINLAND SOCIAL MATURITY SCALE, HE ACHIEVED A MATURITY RATING OF 5.2 YEARS DERIVATING TO A QUOTIENT OF 79. IN THIS AREA HE IS NOT SO UNSKILLED AS HE CARES FOR HIMSELF AT BEDTIME AND AT BATHING AND PLAYS COMPETITIVE EXERCISE GAMES. INTELLECTUALLY, HE HAS SHOWN A RECENT SPURT, ESPECIALLY IN DEVELOPING A VOCABULARY WHICH INCLUDES WORDS AS "GROWN,

Eyelash, and Alligator." Also, he is able to count a few objects and decipher simple mazes. This acceleration now shows him with an I.Q. of 76.

Thus it appears that John's being able to domineer his buddies allows him compensation for his visual handicap (strabismus) as he shows the confident acceleration sometimes shown by an elected leader. At this rate, John will be ready for an educational program shortly, within a year is indicated.

SUMMARY

Chance may have created some of the noticeable dichotomy in the behavior of these twins, however, a true difference in personalities may be evolving due to differences in physical size and visual abilities. Also the social setting, as John's over protectiveness may hinder James by eliciting the reverse.

Careful attention by the nurse and attendants to treat them as individuals and not as a pair seems indicated. Else, John will be ready for school one year and maybe two years ahead of James, leaving James in a lurch only to have to make it up later or to fail.

Virgil B. Sterling
Psychologist
VBS/au

PSYCHOLOGIAL EXAMINATION

DATE: SEPTEMBER 9, 1959

RE-EVALUATION ON THE WISC

JOHN WAS TESTED TODAY WITH THE WECHSLER INTELLIGENCE SCALE FOR CHILDREN TO EVALUATE HIS EDUCATIONAL POTENTIALITY. FOR OVER TWO YEAR, WE HAVE CONSIDERED JOHN AS EDUCABLE AS REFLECTED BY STANFORD-BINET I.Q. RATINGS CONSISTENTLY ABOVE 60.

PRESENT RESULTS ON THE WISC WERE – VERBAL SCALE I.Q. = 80; PERFORMANCE I.Q. = 78 WITH A FULL SCALE I.Q. OF 77. JOHN IS NOW 7 YEARS 7 MONTHS OF AGE WHICH DERIVES TO A MENTAL AGE OF APPROXIMATELY 6 YEARS. BY MOST CRITERIA, THIS WOULD MEAN THAT JOHN IS READY TO BEGIN HIS ACADEMIC TRAINING.

QUALITATIVELY, JOHN IS AN ALERT NEGRO BOY, ONE OF TWINS. HIS GENERAL COMPREHENSION, COUNTING ABILITY AND HIS QUICK WORK WITH PUZZLES ARE HIS BEST AREAS. READING READINESS IS SOMEWHAT BEHIND AS REFLECTED BY A SCALED SCORE OF 2 IN CODING. (HIS AVERAGE SCALED SCORE WAS 7.7) THIS MAY INDICATE A POOR VISUAL-MOTOR COORDINATION WHEN DEALING WITH SYMBOLS; THE HANDICAPPING EFFECT OF HIS STRABISMUS.

HOWEVER, THIS MAY NOT BE TOO LARGE A PROBLEM IN LIGHT OF HIS ALERTNESS. WHEN ASKED HOW BEER AND WINE ARE ALIKE, HE REPLIED "NOT FOR BOYS, THAT'S FOR MEN TO DRINK IT UP." ALSO, BRICK IS BETTER THAN WOOD FOR HOUSES BECAUSE "THEN THE WOLF CAN'T COME AND GET YOU." AND BREAK MEANS "TO GO AWAY AND DRINK COFFEE." THIS LAST DEFINITION SEEMS PECULIARLY CLOSE TO AN INSTITUTION. YET, HE SEEMS READY FOR A SPECIAL EDUCATION PROGRAM TO KEEP HIM COMING ALONG AT A GOOD PACE. HIS MATURITY CONTINUES TO IMPROVE SHOWING HIS FACILITY FOR SELF-DIRECTION

VIRGIL B. STERLING
PSYCHOLOGIST
VBS/AU

RECREATION REPORT

SEPTEMBER 25, 1959

JOHN HAS BEEN IN THE RECREATION PROGRAM FOR ABOUT TWO AND ONE-HALF YEARS. THE PROBLEMS OF BEING WITH A GROUP THAT WAS NOT ON THE LEVEL WITH HIS MENTAL AND PHYSICAL ABILITY HAVE BEEN REMOVED BY HIS BEING TRANSFERRED TO A WARD WHICH CHALLENGES HIS CAPACITY. HE HAS SHOWN REMARKABLE PROGRESS IN THE PROGRAM SINCE HE WAS TRANSFERRED FROM THE TODDLE WARD TO THE TEENAGE WARD.

HE FOLLOWS DIRECTION READILY AND HIS PATIENT RELATIONSHIP IS VERY GOOD. HIS BEHAVIOR IN CLASS IS GOOD. HE HAS ADEQUATE SELF-CARE HABITS AND HIS APPEARANCE IS NEAT. VERBAL COMMUNICATION IS VERY GOOD. HE DISPLAYS A PLEASANT DISPOSITION AT ALL TIMES AND RESPECTS THE AUTHORITY OF THOSE DIRECTING HIM.

IN RECREATIONAL ACTIVITIES HE IS VERY GOOD IN THE FOLLOWING: DANCING, SOCIAL AND SQUARE; SINGING; TUMBLING (EXCEPTIONAL ABILITY) AND BASEBALL. JOHN IS ALSO BEGINNING TO SHOW HIS ABILITY TO SHOULDER RESPONSIBILITIES.

ROBERT T. WOODFORD   (MRS) AMY EVELYN PARKS
RECREATION, AIDE   RECREATION INSTRUCTOR

PSYCHOLOGICAL REPORT

DATE: JUNE 28, 1960

JOHN APPEARS SOMEWHAT DISTRACTIBLE. ALTHOUGH HE WAS FAIRLY COOPERATIVE DURING THE FIRST PART OF THE TEST, HE SOON LOST INTEREST AND BECAME QUITE RESTLESS. IT APPEARS THAT HE DID NOT PERFORM AT THE BEST OF IS ABILITY THROUGHOUT THE TEST, THUS THESE RESULTS POSSIBLY DO NOT REFLECT HIS MAXIMUM LEVEL OF FUNCTIONING.

ON THE REVISED STANFORD-BINET SCALE, FORM L, JOHN EARNED A MENTAL AGE OF 5 YEARS AND 10 MONTHS WITH AN INTELLIGENCE QUOTIENT OF 70, WHICH PLACES HIM IN THE BORDERLINE CLASSIFICATION. HE PASSED ALL IT EMS AT YEAR IV AND HIS SUCCESSES EXTENDED INTO YEAR VIII. BELOW HIS MENTAL AGE LEVEL HE FAILED ITEMS SAMPLING ATTENTION SPAN AND VERBAL COMPREHENSION. HIS HIGHEST SUCCESS WAS ON ITEMS SAMPLING NUMBER CONCEPT.

ACCORDING TO THESE RESULTS, JOHN IS FUNCTIONING AT THE BORDERLINE LEVEL. ONE SUSPECTS THAT, HAD HE PUT FORTH MORE EFFORT, HE COULD HAVE ACHIEVED GREATER SUCCESS ON THIS TEST; HOWEVER, HIS MAXIMUM ABILITY IS PROBABLY WITHIN THE BORDERLINE RANGE.

COLDWATER STATE HOME AND TRAINING SCHOOL

SEPT 5, 1956   RECEIVED AT THE COLDWATER STATE HOME AND TRAINING SCHOOL BY PROBATE COURT COMMITMENT OF KENT COUNTY. BROUGHT FROM HOME OF PATERNAL UNCLE, MR. AND MRS. FRANK PHARMS, 733 CASS SE., GRAND RAPIDS, MICHIGAN, BY MR. ROGER VANEKLASE, JUVENILE PROBATION OFFICER. RECEIVED BY MRS. BRICKLEY. TAKEN TO NURSERY BY MRS. BRICKLEY. OPERATIVE PERMISSION BLANK MAILED TO PROBATE JUDGE. APS.

SEPT 21, 1956   TRANSFERRED TO FORT CUSTER STATE HOME THIS DATE. LH

OCT 30, 1956   VERY ACTIVE, TALKS A GREAT DEAL, AFFECTIONATE. FEEDS SELF. TOILET TRAINED. SH/VEVS

JUNE 6, 1957   DEEP ABRASION APPROXIMATELY 1 INCH LONG ON RIGHT SIDE OF TONGUE. BLEEDING PROFUSE. PRESSURE APPLIED AND ZEPHRIN APPLIED. REPORT ON FILE. EVS.

JUNE 6, 1957   WENT TO THE OPHTHALMOLOGY CLINIC AT THE U OF M HOSPITAL TODAY FOR EVALUATION FOR EYE SURGERY. MB

APRIL 2, 1958   TEST FOR SHIGELLA, NO GROWTH 5-1-58 NOT FOUND

NOV 7, 1958   ENTERIC INFECTIONS, FECES, MICH. DEPT. OF HEALTH – NOT FOUND (NEVER POSITIVE)

NOV 26, 1958	SAME AS ABOVE	NO GROWTH
DEC 4, 1958	SAME AS ABOVE	NO GROWTH
DEC 8, 1958	SAME AS ABOVE (3RD NO GROWTH, NEVER PREVIOUSLY POSITIVE) NO GROWTH	
DEC 17, 1958	SAME AS ABOVE	NO GROWTH
DEC 23, 1958	SAME AS ABOVE	NO GROWTH
DEC 29, 1958	SAME AS ABOVE	NOT FOUND
JAN 8, 1959	SAME AS ABOVE	NOT FOUND

JAN 24, 1959	SAME AS ABOVE	NOT FOUND

SEPT 26, 1959   PA OF CHEST, NO CHANGE – ESSENTIALLY NEGATIVE SAY/MB

DEC 9, 1959   PA OF CHEST; ESSENTIALLY NO CHANGE ALTHOUGH THE MARKINGS MAY BE A LITTLE MORE PROMINENT EXTENDING FROM THE ROOTS OF BOTH LUNGS. I SEE NO DEFINITE PNEUMONITIS PRESENT BUT THE PRESENT FINDINGS WOULD FIT IN WITH BRONCHITIS.

JAN 11, 1960   RECEIVED AT THE COLDWATER STATE AND TRAINING SCHOOL BY ORDER OF TRANSFER FROM FORT CUSTER STATE HOME. BROUGHT BY MR. AND MRS. GETTINGS, ATTENDANTS. RECEIVED BY MRS. HERMAN, TAKEN TO HOSPITAL ADMISSION. AS

JAN 23, 1960   HOSPITAL: ADMITTED FOR TREATMENT U.R.I.

APRIL 16, 1960   HOSPITAL: ADMITTED WITH UPPER RESPIRATORY INFECTION.

APRIL 20, 1960   TRANSFERRED FROM HOSPITAL GENERAL TO ISOLATION WITH MEASLES. SCH.

APRIL 25, 1960   RELEASED FROM HOSPITAL. SCH.

MAY 28, 1960   MEDICAL NOTE: JOHN FELL FROM A SWING AND HIT THE TOP OF HIS HEAD SUSTAINING A ONE-1/2 LACERATION. SEVEN SUTURES REQUIRED. FROM "A" FILED.

JUNE 29, 1960   HOSPITAL: ADMITTED FOR TREATMENT OF BOIL ON THE ANTERIOR SURFACE OF THE NECK. HE IS RECEIVING ANTIBIOTICS AND HOT WET DRESSING. DR. HAMILTON/DL

JULY 1, 1960   RELEASED FROM HOSPITAL. SCH

AUG 18, 1960   PSYCHOLOGICAL REPORT, BY CONSTANCE ELLIGET, FILED IN FOLDER. REVISED STANFORD-BINET SCALE, FROM L; CA 9-6; MA 6-6; IQ 68; HIGH GRADE MORON. IS

Aug 22, 1960	PSYCHOLOGICAL REPORT, BY E.W. GRAY, FILED IN FOLDER. REVISED STANFORD-BINET SCALE, FROM M; CA;10-6; MA 6-10; IQ 65; HIGH GRADE MORON. IS
Jan 1, 1963	HOSPITAL: ADMITTED FOR TREATMENT OF AN UPPER RESPIRATORY INFECTION. DR. GEIB/PL
Jan 7, 1963	RELEASED FROM HOSPITAL. PL
Feb 7, 1963	HOSPITAL: ADMITTED FOR TREATMENT OF RASH OVER HIP. (ISOLATION.) DR. HEINRICH/PL
Feb 8, 1963	MEDICAL NOTE: THE ONLY FINDINGS OF NOTE WERE MILD SWELLING OF THE BURSA OF THE TROCHANT. DR. HEINRICH/PL
July 12, 1963	PSYCHOLOGICAL REPORT, BY CONSTANCE ELLIGET, FILED IN FOLDER. WECHSLER INTELLIGENCE SCALE FOR CHILDREN; CA 11-5; V 62; P 87; F 72; BORDERLINE. IS

COLDWATER STATE HOME AND TRAINING SCHOOL

JUNE, 1963

ACADEMIC   JOHN NEEDS GUIDANCE…HIS READING VOCABULARY HAS EVIDENCE OF

BEING PRIMARY SIGHT, WITH LITTLE PERCEPTION AND PHONETIC

ANALYSIS SKILLS. NOW HE IS HAVING PROBLEMS IN WORD

RECOGNITION…HE HAS STARTED CURSIVE WRITING. MR. KLINE

REPORT OF CONSULTATION

SEPTEMBER 10, 1963

THERE IS A VERY EVIDENT ALTERNATING CONVERGENT STRABISMUS PRESENT. OTHERWISE, THE EYES SEEM NORMAL IN ALL RESPECTS AND PATIENT HAS 20/15; 20/15 VISION AND NO EYE DISCOMFORTS. PATIENT REFERRED FOR POSSIBLE MUSCLE SURGERY BY SURVICAL APPROVAL. ONLY A COSMETIC RESULT COULD BE OBTAINED AND THIS COULD BE UNCERTAIN IN RESULTS AS PATIENT IS NOW ABOUT 11 YEARS OLD. I SEE NO NEED FOR SURGICAL APPROVAL IN THIS CASE UNLESS THE INSTITUTION FEELS IT SHOULD SPEND THE NECESSARY MONEY/EXPENSE TO TRY TO OBTAIN A COSMETIC RESULT.

DR. BIEN, CONSULTING PHYSICIAN

JAN 29, 1964   COLLATERAL INTERVIEW: THE WORKER INTERVIEWS OF BOTH, MR.

**, AND HIS PARENTS DURING THE VISIT TO BATTLE CREEK. IT WAS

RATHER APPARENT THAT THEY HAD ANTICIPATED THAT THE BOYS WERE

BEING CONSIDERED FOR FAMILY CARE, FOR WHEN THE WORKER

MENTIONED THAT FAMILY CARE WAS A POSSIBILITY FOR THE BOYS IN

THE FUTURE, MR. ** STARTED THAT HE UNDERSTOOD THAT THIS WAS

TO HAPPEN. HE CONTINUED, REMARKING THAT HE HAD BEEN INFORMED

THE PREVIOUS YEAR BY MR. FAHLEN THAT THE BOYS WERE TO BE

PLACED, BUT NOTHING HAD HAPPENED. THE WORKER EXPLAINED TO MR.

** THAT IT WOULD BE WISE TO TERMINATE ALL RELATIONS WITH THE

BOYS. HE REMARKED THAT HE HAD BEEN WONDERING WHAT TO DO AS

HE HAD BEEN VERY BUSY. WHETHER MR. ** WAS AFRAID OF THE

WORKER DISCOVERING ANY EVIDENCE OF AN UNHEALTHY RELATIONSHIP

COULD NOT BE DETERMINED FOR CERTAIN, BUT AGREEMENT OVER THE

OBJECT OF THE TRIP HAD BEEN ACCOMPLISHED, THAT OF THE

TERMINATION OF RELATIONSHIP OF MR. ** AND THE PHARMS TWINS.

AXLE.JOHNSON/MR.

JAN 29, 1964   COLLATERAL INTERVIEW: MRS. KNAPP, JOHN'S TEACHER, WAS

VISITED TO DETERMINE HIS BEHAVIOR WHILE IN SCHOOL. MRS. KNAPP

REMARKED THAT SHE WAS CURIOUS WHY THE SOCIAL WORKER WAS

SEEING JOHN, AND QUITE HAPPY THAT MORE COMMUNICATION BETWEEN

THE SOCIAL SERVICES DEPARTMENT AND THE SCHOOL WAS BEING

ESTABLISHED. MRS. KNAPP REMARKED, "JOHN HAS DONE EXTREMELY

WELL IN SCHOOL, ALTHOUGH HE DOES LIKE TO BE THE CENTER OF

ATTENTION AND IS AGGRESSIVE." SHE APPEARED TO HOLD JOHN IN A

VERY HIGH REGARD, REMARKING THAT SHE OFTEN HAD LONG TALKS

WITH HIM ABOUT MANY SUBJECTS.

AXEL JOHNSON/MR

COLDWATER STATE HOME AND TRAINING SCHOOL

JUNE, 1964

ACADEMIC   VERY AGGRESSIVE, DISPLAYING LITTLE TOLERANCE FOR A CONTROLLED

SITUATION OR FOR THE RIGHTS OF OTHERS. WANTS TO BE THE CENTER

OF ATTENTION. DISTRACTIBLE…CANNOT FOLLOW ALONG WITH ANY

DISCUSSION…OFTEN INTERRUPTS. HAS A GREAT DEAL OF DRIVE IF HE IS

IN COMPETITION.

ACADEMIC ACHIEVEMENT:

READING: LEVEL II (COMPREHENSION FAIRLY GOOD)

ARITHMETIC: SAME AS ABOVE

CAN WRITE LETTERS AND STORIES QUITE INDEPENDENTLY…NEEDING

HELP ONLY ON BIGGER WORDS.

MUSIC: TONAL ABILITY: GOOD

WORD MASTERY: LEARNS QUICKLY BUT HIS DICTION MAKES HIM

DIFFICULT TO UNDERSTAND AT TIMES

RHYTHMIC ABILITY: EXCELLENT

BEHAVIOR: JOHN LIKES MUSIC, PARTICULARLY RHYTHMIC

ACTIVITIES AND HAS DONE WELL THIS YEAR. HE

HAS NOW BEEN PLACED ON FAMILY CARE SO IS NO

LONGER IN CLASS. MR. CLARK

PHYS. ED   JOHN IS FAIRLY A WELL DEVELOPED COLORED BOY WHO LIKES ALL

GAMES, IS FAIRLY WELL COORDINATED AND SHOWS FAIR

SPORTSMANSHIP. JOHN GETS ALONG FAIRLY WELL WITH THE GROUP, COOPERATES AND IS FAIRLY DEPENDABLE. THIS BOY HAS MADE BUT LITTLE PROGRESS IN SWIMMING. HIS ENDURANCE WAS ABOVE AVERAGE AND HE SWAM 2200 FEET WITHOUT STOPPING DURING 30 MINUTES. MR. ZEK

FEB 5, 1964   PATIENT INTERVIEW: THE WORKER TOOK JOHN OUT FOR A FIDE ON THIS INTERVIEW, BUYING HIM A HAMBURGER AND MALTED MILK. JOHN APPEARED VERY INTERESTED IN THE BUILDINGS AND LANDMARKS OF THE TOWN. JOHN ASKED MANY QUESTIONS PERTAINING TO THE FUNCTIONING OF INDIVIDUALS ON THE "OUTSIDE." JOHN IS APPARENTLY A CENTER OF ATTENTION IN HIS COTTAGE, HE APPEARED QUITE EMBARRASSED. MANY OF JOHN'S COTTAGE MATES RAN TO THE WORKER AND ASKED ABOUT THEIR GOING ON FAMILY CARE LIKE JOHN. THE WORKER HAS NOT SPECIFICALLY STATED TO JOHN THAT HE WILL GO ON FAMILY CARE, BUT RATHER THAT THERE IS THE POSSIBILITY OF SUCH A MOVE. AXEL JOHNSON/MR

FEB 5, 1964   COLLATERAL INTERVIEW: THE WORKER INTERVIEWED MRS. DOLL, JOHN'S COTTAGE MATRON, UPON RETURNING HIM TO HIS COTTAGE. SHE REMARKED THAT SHE WAS CURIOUS WHY JOHN WAS BEING SEEN BY A SOCIAL WORKER. THE WORKER EXPLAINED TO HER WHY JOHN WAS BEING SEEN. MRS. DOLL REMARKED THAT SHE DIDN'T THINK ANY OF THE BOYS IN COTTAGE 1 WERE CAPABLE OF FUNCTIONING IN FAMILY CARE. SHE STATED THIS IN A VERY SARCASTIC TONE OF VOICE. AXEL JOHNSON/MR

APRIL 4, 1964   PSYCHOLOGICAL REPORT: E.W. GRAY, FILED IN FOLDER. REVISED STANFORD-BINET SCALE, FORM L; CA 12-2; MA 6-8; IQ 55; LOW GRAD MORON. IS

MAR 23, 1864   PATIENT INTERVIEW: IT APPEARED THAT THE PREVIOUS COMBINED INTERVIEW HAD SERVED ITS FUNCTION. JOHN DID NOT QUESTION OR TEST THE WORKER AS HE HAD DONE IN PREVIOUS INTERVIEW. IT IS PROBABLY THAT JOHN HAS FOUND THAT THE WORKER HAS BEEN HONEST WITH BOTH TWINS, AND HAS NOT BEEN DECEIVING THEM. HE WAS QUITE FRIENDLY THROUGHOUT THE INTERVIEW, SMILING CONSTANTLY. A.JOHNSON/MR

APRIL 1, 1964   PATIENT INTERVIEW: JOHN HAS APPARENTLY ACCEPTED THE FACT THAT THE TWINS WILL BE PLACED SEPARATELY, AND THAT JAMES WILL BE PLACED FIRST. HE REMARKED THAT HE WAS GLAD JAMES WAS GOING OUT FIRST. THIS STATEMENT FOLLOWS THE ROLE EXPECTATIONS THAT HAS BEEN ATTRIBUTED TO JOHN, THAT OF THE PARENT. THIS COULD ALSO BE PARTIALLY DUE TO A RATIONALIZATION BY JOHN SO HE WOULD NOT FEEL THAT HE HAD BEEN REJECTED AND JAMES PREFERRED. A. JOHNSON/MR

APRIL 8, 1964   PATIENT INTERVIEW: JOHN WAS QUITE CURIOUS AS TO WHAT HAD TAKEN PLACE WHILE JAMES WAS ON VACATION. IN PREVIOUS INTERVIEWS THE POSSIBILITY OF JAMES LEAVING THE INSTITUTION WAS VERBALIZED, BUT MAY NOT HAVE SEEMED A REALITY TO JOHN. JAMES' GRAND RAPIDS VACATION MAY HAVE MADE THE POSSIBILITY OF LOSING JAMES SEEM MORE REAL, AND CAUSED JOHN TO QUESTION WHEN HE WOULD BE PLACED IN A HOME. THE LONG RANGE GOAL WILL BE TO PLACE JOHN IN A FAMILY CARE HOME. AXEL JOHNSON/MR

MAY 14, 1964   NOTE: DISCUSSED BY COMMITTEE COMPOSED OF DR. WISE, DR. WALTON, DR. GEIB, DR. HEINRICH, MR. HARRIS, MRS. BRADLEY, MISS COX. PLACEMENT IN FAMILY CARE WAS APPROVED. THERE WAS CONSIDERABLE DISCUSSION ABOUT THE SEPARATION OF TWINS, WITH DR. WALTON ASKING THAT HIS VOTE AGAINST SEPARATION BE MADE A MATTER OF RECORD. THE MAJORITY FELT SEPARATION TO BE NECESSARY THIS TIME BUT THAT VISITS SHOULD BE ARRANGED WITH FAIR FREQUENCE, UNDER THE PLAN AS OUTLINED BY SOCIAL SERVICE ALICE L. COX/L.

APRIL 22, 1964   COLLATERAL INTERVIEW: THE WORKER SPOKE WITH MRS. KNAPP ABOUT JOHN'S PROGRESS. SHE STATED THAT HE WAS WELL BEHAVED AND HAD ADVANCED TO THE 3RD GRADE READING LEVEL. SHE EXPRESSED CONCERN OVER THE VALIDITY OF JOHN'S LAST PSYCHOLOGICAL TESTING. SHE STATED THAT SHE KNEW JOHN WAS FUNCTIONING AT A HIGHER LEVEL THAN WAS INDICATED.

MAY 3, 1964   PATIENT INTERVIEW: JOHN WAS RETURNED TO THE INSTITUTION FROM HIS VACATION. WHEN I ARRIVED HE WAS PLAYING BADMINTON WITH CHARLES AND ANDY, PRESENTLY ON FAMILY CARE IN THE ROBINSON HOME, JUST A COUPLE OF DOORS FROM THE DELPHS. JOHN APPEARED QUITE UNHAPPY ABOUT LEAVING THE DELPH HOME AND ASKED ME BEFORE WE LEFT THE HOUSE WHEN WE WOULD RETURN FOR GOOD. THE DELPH'S TOO, APPEARED SAD ABOUT JOHN'S DEPARTURE AND STATED THAT HE CERTAINLY WAS QUITE A NICE YOUNG MAN DURING HIS VISIT. THEY WERE ANXIOUS TO KNOW WHEN HE MIGHT RETURN TO STAY. DURING THE CAR RIDE, JOHN'S CONVERSATION WAS CENTERED AROUND THE DELPH'S AND WHEN HE COULD RETURN THERE. HE REFERRED TO THE DELPHS AS "MOM" AND "DAD", HE MENTIONED HIS "BROTHER," JERRY AND HE EVEN REFERRED TO HIS "NIECE". JOHN WAS NOT PARTICULARLY TALKATIVE AND RESPONDED ONLY TO DIRECT QUESTIONS. HE TRIED WITHOUT SUCCESS, TO PIN ME DOWN ABOUT THE EXACT DATE OF HIS PLACEMENT WITH THE DELPHS ON FAMILY CARE. ON RETURNING TO THE COTTAGE, THE BOYS GREETED JOHN HAPPILY AND, AS I LEFT, JOHN WAS DEEPLY ENGAGED IN CONVERSATION WITH A GROUP OF HIS COTTAGE "PALS".

LINDA SHELLES/BMM.

MAY 20, 1964	PLACED ON FAMILY CARE THIS DATE IN THE HOME OF MR. AND MRS. HENRY DELPH, 936 RUSSELL STREET, JACKSON, MI.
MAY 21, 1964	SUPERVISORY VISIT: JOHN WAS ASSISTING MRS. DELPH IN THE GARDEN WHEN THE WORKER ARRIVED. JOHN SMILED AND LOOKED AS IF HE WERE QUITE PROUD OF BEING ABLE TO ASSIST IN THE GARDEN. JOHN REMARKED TO THE WORKER THAT HE HAD TALKED TO HIS AUNT ON THE TELEPHONE, REFERRING TO MRS. DELPH'S SISTER, AND THAT SHE WAS COMING TO SEE HIM ON THE WEEKEND. JOHN ASKED THE WORKER IF HE WOULD BE SEEING HIM AGAIN. THE WORKER ANSWERED THAT HE'D HAVE ANDY, CHARLES, RICKY AND ALL THE OTHER CHILDREN TO KEEP HIM COMPANY, PLUS HIS MOM AND DAD, SO HE WOULDN'T MISS THE WORKER. THIS APPEARED TO SATISFY HIM AND HE THEN SAID GOOD-BYE. AXEL JOHNSON/BMM
MAY 27, 1964	SUPERVISORY VISIT: JOHN GREETED THE WORKER WITH A BROAD GRIN AND STATED THAT HE WAS GOING TO BECOME A MEMBER OF THE BOY SCOUTS. HE REMARKED THAT THEY WOULD BE GOING ON A CANOE TRIP SOMETIME DURING THE SUMMER. HE APPEARED TO BE VERY PROUD OF BEING ACCEPTED AS A SCOUT. AXEL JOHNSON/BMM
AUG. 3, 1964	COLLATERAL INTERVIEW WITH MR. DAVID BARRETT REGARDING A SCHOOL PLACEMENT FOR JOHN PHARMS. MR. BARRETT WAS INFORMED THAT JOHN WOULD ATTEND TOMLINSON SCHOOL. FOR ENROLLMENT, JOHN WILL NEED A RECORD OF IMMUNIZATION AND SOME PROOF OF HIS BIRTH DATE. SCHOOL BEGINS SEPTEMBER 9, AT WHICH TIME HE CAN REGISTER BY GOING TO THE PRINCIPAL'S OFFICE.

The Untold Yet Remarkable Story of a Very Determined Little Boy Named Johnnie

L. SHELLES/MB

PSYCHOLOGIAL REPORT

RETEST

MAY 12, 1967

JOHN HAS GROWN INTO A ROBUST, VERY OUTGOING BOY WHO MOVED RESTLESSLY DURING THE TEST, EXPRESSING DISGUST WITH THE EASY ITEMS AND BECOMING VERY SOLEMN WHEN THE PROBLEMS WERE DIFFICULT. IN GENERAL, COOPERATION SEEMED GOOD, HOWEVER, WITH JOHN REMARKING CANDIDLY, AND WITH FAIR ACCURACY, ON THE QUALITY OF HIS ANSWERS. TOWARD THE END OF THE PROCEDURE, HE WAS INCREASINGLY RESTLESS, PROBABLY DUE TO THE RELATIVE INACTIVITY, HIS RESPONSES WERE OFFERED WITH HURRIED CARELESSNESS.

THE **WESCHLER INTELLIGENCE SCALE FOR CHILDREN** WAS ADMINISTERED. LOW VERBAL SCORES EMPHASIZED A NARROW RANGE OF GENERAL INFORMATION AND A LIMITED VOCABULARY. COMPREHENSION, JUDGEMENT AND REASONING WERE RELATIVELY GOOD, WITH ADEQUATE, THOUGH SOMEWHAT SUPERFICIAL UNDERSTANDING OF WORD AND CONCEPT RELATIONSHIPS. PERFORMANCE SCORES PRIMARILY REVEALED AVERAGE NON-VERBAL ABILITY. SPATIAL PERCEPTION, AS MEASURED ON THE RELATIVELY ABSTRACT BLOCK DEIGN TEST, FELL SOMEWHAT BELOW THE MORE CONCRETE ORGANIZATIONAL PROBLEMS. PRESENT RESULTS:

CHRONOLOGICAL AGE	:	15 YEARS, 3 MONTHS
VERBAL SCALE I.Q.	: 76	
PERFORMANCE SCALE I.Q.	: 92	
FULL SCALE I.Q.	: 82	
CLASSIFICATION	:	BORDERLINE

JOHN ATTENDS SCHOOL, STATES THAT HE IS IN THE EIGHTH GRADE AND IS ACTIVE IN SPORTS. A VERY FRIENDLY BOY, AND FAIRLY ALERT, HE SHOULD CONTINUE TO PROGRESS SATISFACTORILY.

CONSTANCE ELLIGET/IS

TYPED MAY 16, 1967

AUG. 31, 1964   SUPERVISORY VISIT: JOHN SEEMS TO HAVE ADJUSTED QUITE WELL TO THE FAMILY SITUATION, AND THE DELPHS ENJOY HAVING HIM PARTICIPATE IN THEIR ACTIVITIES. JOHN ASKED ABOUT JIM AND HE WANTS JIM TO COME AND STAY WITH HIM IN JACKSON. ALTHOUGH JOHN DID NOT SEE JIM MUCH AT THE INSTITUTION, HE INFORMS ME THAT HE MISSES HIM. JOHN DIDN'T SEEM TO HEAR THE STATEMENT ABOUT OUR NOT KNOWING JIM WELL ENOUGH, BUT HE DID STATE THAT JIM TALKED TO HIM WHEN HE SAW HIM THERE. THROUGHOUT OUR INTERVIEW THE ONLY CONVERSATION THAT JOHN CARED TO CARRY ON ABOUT WAS CONVERSATION ABOUT JIM COMING TO JACKSON TO STAY WITH HIM. HE IS QUITE ANXIOUS FOR SCHOOL, ESPECIALLY BOY SCOUTS, TO BEGIN. MRS. DELPH MENTIONED THAT JOHN TALKS ABOUT JIM A LOT, AND IT APPEARS THAT MRS. DELPH AND JOHN MAY BE ATTEMPTING TO EFFECT JIM'S PLACEMENT HERE.

SEPT. 22, 1964   COLLATERAL VISIT: WITH MR. MOORE, TEACHER AT ALLEN SCHOOL. MR. MOORE INFORMED THAT, THUS FAR, JOHN HAS PRESENTED NO DIFFICULTIES IN THE CLASSROOM. HE STATED THAT HE WOULD APPRECIATE ANY INFORMATION WE CAN PROVIDE HIM ABOUT JOHN, SO THAT HE CAN MAKE JOHN'S PROGRAM MORE SUITABLE TO HIS NEEDS. I STATED THAT INFORMATION WOULD BE SENT TO HIM ABOUT JOHN AT AN EARLY AGE.

NOV. 30, 1964   SUPERVISORY VISIT: JOHN WAS IN SCHOOL AND MRS. DELPH INFORMED, THAT IN GENERAL, JOHN CONTINUES HIS ADJUSTMENT SATISFACTORILY. LAST WEEK, HOWEVER, MR. MOORE, JOHN'S SCHOOL TEACHER, SENT A NOT HOME WITH JOHN, STATING THAT JOHN HAS BEEN SASSY IN THE CLASSROOM AND HAD REFUSED TO DO WHAT HE WAS

ASKED TO DO. MR. & MRS. DELPH HANDLED THIS WITH JOHN AND HE APPARENTLY HAS NOT BEEN IN TROUBLE SINCE THEN. MRS. DELPH WAS ABLE TO CITE OTHER WAYS IN WHICH JOHN HAD PROGRESSED SINCE HIS PLACEMENT THERE. FOR EXAMPLE, JOHN WAS EXTREMELY TALKATIVE AND MENTIONED QUITE OFTEN HIS VISITS WITH MR. ** IN BATTLE CREEK. NOW, HOWEVER, JOHN ALMOST NEVER MENTIONS MR. ** AND TALKS IN A MORE APPROPRIATE MANNER. HE HASN'T LOST ANY OF HIS ENTHUSIASM FOR BOY SCOUTS AND HE HAS NOW WORKED UP TO A FIRST CLASS SCOUT RATING. MRS. DELPH SPEAKS QUITE FONDLY OF JOHN AND SHE EVIDENCES AN INTEREST IN JOHN'S ACTIVITIES. SHE HAS VISITED THE SCHOOL AND SEEMS TO HAVE MADE SATISFACTORY CONTACTS WITH JOHN'S TEACHERS.

SHELLES/JR

DEC. 21, 1964   SUPERVISORY VISITS: JOHN IS OUT OF SCHOOL FOR CHRISTMAS VACATION AND WAS PLAYING WITH SOME OF OF HIS NEIGHBORHOOD PALS ACROSS THE STREET. HE CAME TO GREET ME, HOWEVER, AND TO ASK ME TO SAY HI TO JIM.

L. SHELLES/JR

JAN 18, 1965   TELEPHONE CALL TO MRS. DELPH REGARDING LETTERS OF 1/11/65 AND 1/13/65 FROM JOHN'S TEACHER AND PRINCIPAL. MR. DELPH KNEW NOTHING ABOUT MR. MOORE'S INTEREST IN GETTING JOHN AND JAMES TOGETHER, BUT SHE WAS AWARE OF HIS CONCERN REGARDING GETTING HIS EYES STRAIGHTENED. TO MY INQUIRY REGARDING JOHN'S CONTACTS WITH MR. MOORE OUTSIDE SCHOOL, MRS. DELPH SAID ON ONE OCCASION MR. MOORE, WHO UNMARRIED, PREPARED DINNER FOR CHARLES AND JOHN IN THE HOME OF HIS LANDLADY, AND TOOK JOHN

DOWNTOWN SHOPPING ONCE DURING CHRISTMAS VACATION. SHE SAID "HE THINKS JOHN DOESN'T HAVE ANYTHING, BUT HE HAS A HOME HERE AND KEEPS BUSY WITH HIS FRIENDS AND MY SISTER'S SONS." HE SELDOM TALKS ABOUT JAMES NOW.

NELLIE H. LOOMIS/MB

MAR. 12, 1965   SUPERVISORY CALL: JOHN WAS IN SCHOOL, BUT MRS. DELPH SPEAKS PROUDLY OF HIS PROGRESS. HE DOES HIS CHORE WILLINGLY, AND CAN READ THE NEWSPAPER WITH COMPREHENSION. HE IS APPLYING HIMSELF TO HIS STUDIES IN HOPE OF BEING ABLE TO ATTEND JUNIOR HIGH NEXT YEAR WITH CHARLES AND ANDY. ON HIS BIRTHDAY FEB. 21, THEY HAD A PARTY AND INVITED THE BOYS FROM THE ** HOME. THEY GAVE JOHN A TRANSISTOR RADIO. THE COUNTY NURSE HAS ARRANGED FOR JOHN TO SEE THE EYE DOCTOR AT 10:30 A.M. ON MAY 24; DR. KOBS, 120 FRANKLIN STREET. JOHN IS PLEASED TO KNOW THAT THERE IS A POSSIBILITY OF CORRECTING HIS EYE CONDITION.

NELLIE H. LOOMIS/L

JULY 9, 1965   MEDICAL NOTE: AFTER TELEPHONE DISCUSSIONS WITH THE OFFICE OF DR. R. J. KOBS, 120 FRANKLIN STREET, JACKSON…AND WITH MR. PAUL CAVANGH, MCCC, JOHN WAS AUTHORIZED TO ENTER FOOTE HOSPITAL ON JULY 13 FOR EYE SURGERY BY DR. KOBS ON JULY 14.

NELLIE H. LOOMIS/M

JULY 20, 1965   SUPERVISORY VISIT: JOHN, ALONG WITH THE BOYS FOR MRS. ** HOME, PLUS SEVERAL OTHER NEIGHBORHOOD BOYS WERE OUT PLAYING BALL IN THE VACANT LOT WHEN WORKER ARRIVED. JOHN, CHARLES, AND ANDY RECOGNIZED THE STATE CAR AND CAME OUT TO GREET ME. JOHN REPORTED THAT THE ONLY HAD TO REMAIN IN THE HOSPITAL FOR TWO DAYS AFTER EYE SURGERY, AND WAS FEELING FINE. WORKER HAD NEVER MET JOHN BEFORE BUT ASSUMED FROM HAVING READ PATIENT'S RECORD, THAT THE SURGERY HAD DONE MUCH TO IMPROVE HIS APPEARANCE. WORKER MENTIONED THAT SHE WOULD LIKE TO GO MEET HIS MOTHER (MRS. DELPH) AND HE REPLIED THAT "SHE WAS WORKING".

WHEN QUESTIONED AS TO WHETHER SHE WAS HELPING AT SCHOOL, JOHN MENTIONED THAT SHE IS EMPLOYED OUTSIDE THE HOME. THIS SITUATION WILL BE INVESTIGATED. MRS. **, HER NEIGHBOR, WAS APPARENTLY WATCHING JOHN AS HE WAS ENGAGED IN THE BALL GAME WITH HER TWO PATIENTS. AS WORKER WAS LEAVING, JOHN ASKED ABOUT HIS TWIN BROTHER, JAMES. HE WAS SURPRISED TO FIND THAT JAMES WAS ALSO IN FAMILY CARE NOW. HE WANTED TO KNOW HIS ADDRESS SO THAT HE COULD WRITE TO HIM. WORKER SAID SHE WOULD CHECK AND ADVISE HIM ON HER NEXT VISIT.

M. HAZZARD/EP

OCT 12, 1965

SUPERVISORY VISIT: MRS. DELPH KNEW WORKER WAS COMING AND HAD PURPOSELY STAYED HOME TO TALK TO HER BECAUSE SHE HAD BEEN AWAY THE LAST TIME I CALLED. SHE HAD SOME CLOTHES OF JOHN'S; ONE PAIR OF PANTS PRACTICALLY NEW; THAT SHE WAS RETURNING BECAUSE HE HAD GROWN SO FAST THAT A LOT OF THE CLOTHING SHE HAD ORDERED LATE IN THE SUMMER WAS TOO SMALL. HE IS VERY HAPPY IN SCHOOL, AND REALLY ENJOYS FOOTBALL. THEY DON'T EAT UNTIL LATE NOW BECAUSE HE DOESN'T ARRIVE HOME UNTIL SX-THIRTY OR SEVEN IN THE EVENING. HE HAS HAD AN APPOINTMENT WITH DR. KOBS WHO HOPES TO SET UP A SECOND OPERATION ON JOHN'S EYES DURING CHRISTMAS VACATION. WORKER HAD TALKED TO DR. KOBS EARLIER AND HE TOO HAD MENTIONED MORE SURGERY. HE ALSO TOLD ME THAT JOHN WAS A VERY NICE BOY.

M. HAZZARD/MB

JUNE 17, 1966

SUPERVISORY VISIT: I MET JOHN FOR THE FIRST TIME. HE IS A TALL BOY FOR HIS 14 YEARS AND HAS A LARGE FRAME. JOHN SEEMED VERY

FRIENDLY AND WITH A LITTLE URGING SHOWED ME HIS TRACT RIBBONS HE HAS WON IN SCHOOL. MRS. DELPH BROUGHT OUT HIS REPORT CARD. HE RECEIVED AN OVERALL GRADE OF 2.4, WITH TWO "C+'S", ONE "C-", AND THREE "B-'S". JOHN MENTIONED THAT CHARLES WAS ACROSS THE STREET, SO I HAD HIM INTRODUCE ME TO CHARLES AND ANDY WHO WAS SITTING ON THE ** FRONT PORCH. JOHN SEEMS TO HAVE GOOD MANNERS AND INTRODUCED ME FORMALLY AND PROPERLY. HE SAID HE PLANNED ON PLAYING A LOT OF BALL THIS SUMMER.

BLALOCK/AB

SEPT. 7, 1966	SUPERVISORY CALL: JOHN CAME OUT OF THE HOUSE TO GREET WORKER. HE THEN BEGAN TALKING ABOUT SPORTS AND SAID PLANNED TO GO OUT FOR FOOTBALL. HE SAID MR. YOUNG WILL BE HIS COACH AND HE WILL ALSO HAVE HIM FOR A TEACHER FOR TWO OF HIS CLASSES. JOHN IS IN THE 8TH GRADE, SPECIAL EDUCATION PROGRAM. HE HAS A FINE ATTITUDE TOWARD SCHOOL AND OTHERS, AND HE HAS VERY GOOD MANNERS.

B. BLALOCK/AB

OCT. 6, 1966	SUPERVISORY CALL: MRS. DELPH STATED THAT JOHN WAS IN SCHOOL AND THAT HE IS PROUDLY PARTICIPATING ON THE 8TH GRADE FOOTBALL TEAM. SHE REPORTED THAT HE WOULD PROBABLY NOT GET HOME UNTIL ABOUT 6 OR 6:30 P.M. DUE TO HIS FOOTBALL PRACTICE AT SCHOOL.

B. BLALOCK/AB

OCT. 13, 1966	COLLATERAL INTERVIEW WITH MR. DINEHART, ASSISTANT PRINCIPAL OF EAST INTERMEDIATE JUNIOR HIGH SCHOOL IN JACKSON, AND WITH MRS. BORHAM, ONE OF JOHN'S TEACHERS WHO TEACHES

ENGLISH, AND VOCATIONAL GUIDANCE. MR. DINEHART IS VERY

COOPERATIVE AND STATED JOHN CONTINUES TO HAVE A FFINE ATTITUDE

TOWARD SCHOOL AND HAS CREATED NO DISCIPLINE PROBLEMS WHAT-

SO-EVER. HE TOOK ME TO MRS. BORHAM'S ROOM AND INTRODUCED US.

MRS. BORHAM IS AN ATTRACTIVE NEGRO WHO APPEARS TO BE IN HER

EARLY THIRTIES. SHE THOROUGHLY IMPRESSED THIS WORKER WITH HER

UNDERSTANDING, INSIGHT, AND EMPATHY WHICH WAS INDICATED BY

HER THROUGH HER COMMENTS ABOUT JOHN AND HER OTHER STUDENTS

SHE STATED THAT SHE FELT JOHN WAS A VERY SOCIABLE AND

"OUTGOING" BOY WITH "A SMILE FOR EVERYONE." SHE SAID THAT JOHN

HAS TALKED ABOUT HIS MOTHER "NOT WANTING HIM AND HIS BROTHER

JAMES, BUT HE DOESN'T SAY THIS WITH ANY KIND OF HOSTILITY, BUT

RATHER MATTER OF FACTLY." MRS. BARHAM REPORTED THAT

SOMETIMES SHE TAKES HER CUE FROM THE STUDENTS AS TO WHAT WILL

BE DISCUSSED. FOR EXAMPLE, SHE SAID ONE MORNING A STUDENT

BOUGHT UP THE SUBJECT OF SEEING A DOG "ON TOP OF ANOTHER DOG",

WHICH MRS. BARHAM DEVELOPED INTO A DISCUSSION OF MENTAL AND

PHYSICAL HYGIENE AND SEX. SHE STATED THAT IT CAME OUT IN THIS

DISCUSSION THAT "JOHN THOUGHT HUMAN INFANTS (BABIES) WERE

"HATCHED" BY THE MOTHER LIKE AN EGG." SHE FELT THAT SINCE MOST

OF THE STUDENTS WERE QUITE IGNORANT REGARDING SEXUAL

EDUCATION THAT A CLASS SHOULD BE PLANNED FOR THIS SUBJECT.

SUBSEQUENTLY, A MALE TEACHER, MR. YOUNG, WHO MRS. BARHAM

PRAISES AS AN EXCELLENT SPECIAL EDUCATION TEACHER, TOOK ALL OF

THE BOYS IN A CLASS AND SHE TOOK ALL OF THE GIRLS AND HAD A

"REAL GOOD DISCUSSION OF THE BIRDS AND THE BEES." SHE ATTRIBUTES

HER ABILITY TO DO THIS, TO BEING FLEXIBLE IN THE CURRICULUM, TO THE FACT THAT THE PRINCIPAL AND OTHER SCHOOL OFFICIALS AT EAST JUNIOR HIGH URGE THEIR TEACHERS TO BE CREATIVE AND INTERESTING TO THE STUDENTS.

B. BLALOCK/AB

Nov. 8, 1966   SUPERVISORY CALL: MRS. DELPH SHOWED ME THAT SHE IS GIVING JOHN MORE DISCIPLINE THAN WAS THOUGHT IN THE PAST, BY SAYING THAT ONE MORNING HE CAME DOWN WITH A PAIR OF PANTS ON WHICH WERE TOO SHORT AND SHE MADE HIM CHANGE THEM, AND HE DID. BUT HE CAME DOWNSTAIRS WITH A SHIRT THAT HAD NUMEROUS HOLES IN IT AND SHE MADE HIM CHANGE THAT TOO. JOHN DOES MIND WELL, AS IS ILLUSTRATED ABOVE. THE FOOTBALL SEASON IS OVER FOR HIM BUT MRS. DELPH SAID THAT HE HAS BOY SCOUT MEETING EVERY MONDAY EVENING.

B. BLALOCK/DEC

Dec. 15, 1966   COLLATERAL INTERVIEWS WITH MRS. BARHAM AND WITH MR. YOUNG, SPECIAL EDUCATION TEACHERS, WHO HAVE BOTH JOHN AND CHARLES IN ONE OF THEIR CLASSES. BOTH MR. YOUNG AND MRS. BARHAM FELT THAT JOHN SHOULD PARTICIPATE IN MORE ACTIVITIES BOTH AT HOME AND AT SCHOOL. THEY FELT THAT JOHN IS "IMMATURE AND NAIVE." WHEN ASKED BY THE WORKER WHAT THEY SPECIFICALLY MEANT BY THIS, THEY STATED THAT JOHN DIDN'T SEEM AWARE OF SUBTLETIES THAT OCCUR IN REAL LIFE. THEY FEEL THAT THIS WILL BE TO JOHN'S DISADVANTAGE AFTER HE GETS OUT OF SCHOOL. THEY BOTH FEEL THAT JOHN IS PROGRESSING VERY WELL ACADEMICALLY AND THAT HE TRIES VERY HARD. THEY SUGGESTED THAT PERHAPS HIS EYES NEED

EXAMINING AGAIN SINCE THEY HAVE NOTICED THAT AT TIMES HIS EYES APPEAR TO CROSS. THEY STATED THAT HE ALWAYS COME TO SCHOOL CLEAN AND WELL DRESSED.

R. BLALOCK/FE

JAN. 24, 1967   MRS. BARHAM EXPLAINED THAT JOHN'S GRADES HAVE GONE DOWN THIS SEMESTER IN ENGLISH BECAUSE "JOHN TRIES TO FINISH HIS WORK FIRST AND THUS HE DOES NOT TAKE TIME TO DO A GOOD JOB." SHE SAID SHE WOULD WORK WITH HIM ON THIS TO TRY TO GET HIM TO SEE THAT BETTER RESULTS, AND NOT JUST SPEED, WILL DETERMINE HIS GRADES AND PROGRESS. MR. YOUNG HAS JOHN ON HIS BASKETBALL TEAM. HE SAYS JOHN HAS "GOOD" COORDINATION AND "GREAT DESIRE" TO DO GOOD. JOHN REPORTEDLY LOVES BASKETBALL AND MOST SPORTS.

B. BLALOCK/FA

MAR. 7, 1967   COLLATERAL INTERVIEW WITH MR. JOHN YOUNG, ONE OF JOHN'S
                   SPECIAL EDUCATION TEACHERS. MR. YOUNG REPORTED THAT JOHN
                   SEEMS TO BE DRESSING BETTER NOW FOR SCHOOL AND THAT HE SEEMS
                   TO HAVE SOME SMALL CHANGE ON HIM MOST OF THE TIME. MR. YOUNG
                   IS ALSO JOHN'S BASKETBALL COACH AND HE FEELS JOHN HAS A REAL
                   GOOD ATTITUDE TOWARD THE OTHER PLAYERS AND VERY GOOD
                   SPORTSMANSHIP CONDUCT DURING THE GAMES. HE SAID JOHN IS
                   USUALLY THE FIRST ONE TO INITIATE ENTHUSIASM AND ENCOURAGE THE
                   OTHER PLAYER TO WIN.
                   B. BLALOCK/MB

APRIL 25, 1967   SUPERVISORY CALL: JOHN WAS IN SCHOOL, BUT MRS. DELPH
                   REPORTED THAT HE SEEMS TO BE DOING BETTER IN SCHOOL SINCE HIS
                   GRADES HAVE BEEN RAISED SINCE LAST SEMESTER. JOHN IS REPORTEDLY
                   VERY ENTHUSED ABOUT RUNNING IN HIS SCHOOL'S TRACK PROGRAM
                   AND HE REPORTEDLY PRACTICES AFTER SCHOOL EACH NIGHT GETTING
                   HOME ABOUT 5:30 OR 6 P.M. WORKER INFORMED MRS. DELPH THAT HE
                   WOULD PICK UP ON FRIDAY, MAY 12 TO TRANSPORT HIM TO
                   COLDWATER TO PURCHASE SOME GLASS FRAMES FOR HIM
                   B. BLALOCK/MB

MAY 12, 1967   PSYCHOLOGICAL REPORT, BY CONSTANCE ELLIGET FILED IN
                   FOLDER. WECHSLER INTELLIGENCE SCALE FOR CHILDREN: CA 15-3; V
                   76; P 92; F 82: BORDERLINE. IS

JUNE 9, 1967   COLLATERAL INTERVIEW WITH MR. YOUNG, ONE OF JOHN'S
                   SPECIAL EDUCATION TEACHERS. HE STATED THAT JOHN SEEMS TO HAVE
                   PROGRESSED BOTH ACADEMICALLY AND SOCIALLY, STATING THAT JOHN
                   "ALWAYS HAS A SMILE FOR EVERYONE." MR. YOUNG AGREED TO SEND A

WRITTEN EVALUATION OF JOHN'S PROGRESS IN SCHOOL TO MEA AT THE END OF THE SCHOOL YEAR. HE INDICATED THAT THE SPECIAL EDUCATION CLASSES PROBABLY WOULDN'T HAVE ANY ATHLETIC TEAMS NEXT YEAR DUE TO LACK OF SUFFICIENT FUNDS, AS THE MILLAGE INCREASE WAS VOTED DOWN. JOHN IS REPORTEDLY WEARING HIS GLASSES IN SCHOOL EVERY DAY.

B. BLALOCK/MB

Oct. 20, 1967   SUPERVISORY CALL: JOHN WAS HOME SINCE THERE WAS NO SCHOOL THIS DATE. HE SEEMED VERY PROUD OF THE FACT THAT HE WAS PLAYING ON THE 8TH GRADE FOOTBALL TEAM AS AN END. HE LOVES TO TALK SPORTS AND IS VERY "UP" ON THE IN-SEASON SPORTS. JOHN REPORTED THAT HE HAS A JOB AT SCHOOL FOR ONE HOUR EACH DAY. THIS JOB WAS OFFERED TO HIM SINCE HE HAS A "FREE CLASS PERIOD" DURING THE LAST HOUR OF SCHEDULED CLASSES. JOHN SAYS HE IS GETTING $1.25 PER HOUR IN THE SCHOOL CAFETERIA AND CLEANING BLACKBOARDS. JOHN SAYS HE IS DOING BETTER ACADEMICALLY, HAVING RECEIVED ONLY ONE "D" THE FIRST MAKING PERIOD. THE "D" REPORTED IS IN A "SOCIAL SCIENCE" CLASS TAUGHT BY MR. YOUNG – WHO IS ALSO JOHN'S FOOTBALL COACH. JOHN ADMITS TO "MISSING SOME TACKLES" BY RUSHING INTO THE LINE TOO FAST AND BEING OFF-BALANCE.

B. BLALOCK/AB

Nov. 2, 1967   COLLATERAL INTERVIEW WITH MR. FORTRESS, PRINCIPAL OF EAST JR. HIGH SCHOOL AND MR. YOUNG, ON OF JOHN'S TEACHERS. MR. FORTRESS STATED THE "JOHN IS A CREDIT TO THE SCHOOL IN THAT HE HAS A GOOD ATTITUDE TOWARD SCHOOL AND IS TEACHERS, AND HE IS FRIENDLY TO EVERYONE." MR. YOUNG FEELS JOHN IS READING BETTER

THIS YEAR AND NOTED THAT HE LIKES TO READ BOOKS ABOUT SPORTS AS WELL AS AUTOBIOGRAPHIES ABOUT FAMOUS PEOPLE IN SPORTS. MR. YOUNG STATED THAT JOHN WAS MADE CO-CAPTAIN OF THE 8TH GRADE FOOTBALL TEAM AND THAT JOHN IS VERY PROUD OF THIS. AS A CO-CAPTAIN JOHN LEADS THE TEAM IN THE INITIAL CALISTHENICS IN PRACTICES AND BEFORE EACH GAME. JOHN IS SAID TO HAVE A "GUNG-HO" SPIRIT AND IS THE FIRST TO SAY "COME ON YOU GUYS, WE CAN DO BETTER THAN THIS." IN AN INTERVIEW WITH JOHN, HE EXPRESSED MUCH PRIDE AND HUMILITY IN HIS SPORTS ACTIVITIES. IT WAS ALSO LEARNED THAT THE "D" MARK (AS NOTED ON 10/20/67) JOHN SAID RECEIVED IN SOCIAL STUDIES CLASS WAS JUST ON ONE PAPER AND THAT MR. YOUNG FEELS JOHN IS CAPABLE OF RECEIVING A MUCH BETTER MARK AT THE END OF THE SEMESTER. WORKER NOTICED THAT JOHN WAS WEARING A WHITE SHIRT AND TIE UNDERNEATH HIS SCHOOL SWEATER. HE HAD FOOTBALL LETTER AND OTHER EMBLEMS SEWN ON THE SWEATER. HE LOOKED VERY WELL DRESSED FOR SCHOOL. HE SEEMS TO HAVE FINE RAPPORT WITH HIS TEACHER, MR. YOUNG.

B. BLALOCK/ML

JAN. 19, 1968   COLLATERAL INTERVIEW WITH ONE OF JOHN'S TEACHERS, MRS. BARHAM, AT EAST JUNIOR HIGH SCHOOL. JOHN HAS HER FOR SOCIAL STUDIES AND ENGLISH CLASSES. MRS. BARHAM IS QUITE FAMILIAR WITH JOHN, HAVING HAD HIM AS A STUDENT I ONE OF HER CLASSES FOR THE PAST TWO SCHOOL YEARS. SHE REPORTS THAT JOHN IS DOING WELL IN SCHOOL, BUT NEEDS THE GREATEST HELP IN "READING COMPREHENSION." SHE FEELS HE CAN READ WELL (ON APPROX. 5TH GRADE LEVEL), BUT HE READS WORDS TOO FAST AND DOES NOT "GET"

THE MEANING OF THE SENTENCE OR PARAGRAPH. SHE SAYS, HOWEVER, HE DOES LIKE TO READ. WORKER SUGGESTED THAT PERHAPS WE CAN CALL HIS ATTENTION TO POSSIBLY SUBSCRIBING TO A MAGAZINE AND HAVING IT PUT IN HIS NAME , AS WELL AS HAVING HIM SAVE UP FOR THIS OUT HIS ALLOWANCE MONEY SO THAT THIS WOULD HAVE MORE MEANING FOR HIM. JOHN NOW TRIES TO USE HIS INGRATIATING SMILE TO HIS ADVANTAGE IN THE CLASSROOM. FOR EXAMPLE, JOHN "LOVES TO TALK" AND MRS. BARHAM SAID SOMETIMES IT WILL TAKE HER TWO OR THREE TIMES OF ASKING HIM TO STOP TALKING BEFORE HE WILL DO SO BECAUSE HE WILL SMILE AND SAY SOMETHING OR START TO SAY SOMETHING BEFORE SHE IS THROUGH SAYING "STOP TALKING." HE HAS A DISARMING MANNER AND SEEMS O BE DEVELOPING THIS TO HIS ADVANTAGE. MR. FORTRESS, PRINCIPAL, FEELS AGAIN THAT JOHN IS A REAL CREDIT TO THE SCHOOL.

B. BLALOCK/ML

APRIL 11, 1968 …JOHN INDICATED THAT HE IS IN TRAINING FOR THE SCHOOL TRACK TEAM, BUT THAT HIS FAVORITE SPORT IS FOOTBALL. HE HOPES TO MAKE THE VARSITY FOOTBALL TEAM AS A SOPHOMORE NEXT FALL. JOHN PERHAPS HAS UNREALISTIC GOALS IN SPORTS AND ACADEMICALLY FOR THE FUTURE IN THAT HE WANTS TO EARN AN ATHLETIC SCHOLARSHIP TO "A BIG TEN SCHOOL." ACADEMIC ACHIEVEMENT AND GREAT COORDINATION WERE POINTED OUT TO JOHN AS PREREQUISITES FOR COLLEGE AND HADN'T WE BETTER THINK IN TERMS OF WHAT HE CAN DO RATHER THAN JUST WHAT HE WOULD LIKE TO DO. HE ALSO THOUGHT THAT PERHAPS HE WOULD LIKE TO STUDY TO BE AN EDITOR OF A NEWSPAPER. HOWEVER, HE DOES NOT SEEM TO KNOW WHAT THIS

ENCOMPASSES OTHER THAN DEBATING AND DISCUSSING THE "NEWS WITH PEOPLE." JOHN SAYS HE ENJOYS THE "FREE SPEECH HOUR" HE HAS IN SOME OF HIS CLASSES WHERE THE STUDENTS GET TO DISCUSS WHATEVER THEY WANT. JOHN NEEDS MORE HELP IS REALIZING HIS ABILITIES AND APTITUDES. PERHAPS THE WORKER CAN CONSULT WITH JOHN'S TEACHERS AGAIN TO GET THEIR FEELINGS AS TO HOW MUCH JOHN IS THINKING HE CAN AND CAN'T DO IN REGARD TO ACTUAL ABILITIES.

B. BLALOCK/MB

June 18, 1968   …John was proud of his certificates he received for participation in
football, track and basketball. He very proudly stated that their junior high
team, of which he was a starter, won 22 games, including the city
tournament. He also received a certificate for a good job in assisting in the
Science Lab, for which he was paid. He received another school certificate
for having a perfect "attendance record." He said he would have received
a certificate in the 7th and 8th grades but me missed on e and a half days
respectively during the year…John does appear to have a great deal of
confidence in himself and perhaps a bit over-confident, unrealistically. For
example, he has mentioned that he would like to attend college and
perhaps be a professional ball player. It is not clear yet to the worker
whether this is good adolescent idealism or entirely over-confidence in
himself and his abilities. John is very "wrapped up in sports", as many
teenagers his age are, and his real wants or wishes should soon be
crystallizing into realistic thinking……

B. Blalock/ml

Aug. 26, 1968   SOCIAL SERVICE NOTE: ..During the trips to and from Three Rivers,
John conducted himself appropriately in that he discussed his favorite
subject, sports, and responded to conversation by the worker and initiated
it. John still, I feel, has an over-estimate of his athletic and intellectual
prowess. We discussed this in relationship to his current thinking and
future ideas. He has talked about getting an athletic scholarship to college.
Worker pointed out to him realistically, yet not degrading him, that he is
currently in Special Education classes where he is perhaps receiving much
more academic instructional help from his teachers and even now is for
the most part receiving only "C's" and that if he is placed in a regular

classroom he may not receive this much assistance plus the fact that he will have much more academic competition. I indicated that we will continue to talk about his desires and wishes as he progresses on through high school but reminded him that we will more than likely have to lower our sights as to a future job or advanced schooling from a sports announcer to vocational job training…

B. Blalcok/ml

Nov. 21, 1968 …(Mrs. Delph) also gave the worker the parents copy of John's school academic report of 10/16/68 which will be filed in his folder. John received a "C+" in Social Studies; a "B+" in Math; an "A-" in Science and a "B" in English. These are all "10th grade" Special Education classes.

B. Blalock/an

Feb. 25, 1969 SOCIAL SERVICE SUPERVISORY CALL: John was not seen on this date since he was in school. Mrs. Delph gave the worker the "parent copy" of John's academic attendance and citizenship report card, which will be filed in John's folder. John received third semester Special Education grades – 3 "B's"; 1 "C"; and 1 "A". The "B's" were in English, Science and Math and the "C" in Social Studies and the "A" in Speech. John has three different teachers for his five subjects. Mrs. Delph stated that she recently attended one of the 10th grade basketball games, of which John is a starter, playing center. John reportedly is in good health again.

B. Blalock/mb

MAR. 12, 1969   MRS. DELPH SENT THE WORKER A COPY OF JOHN'S REPORT CARD DATED 3/7/69. JOHN MAINTAINED A 3.0 AVERAGE. REFER TO THE "PARENT COPY" OF THE REPORT FILED IN JOHN'S FOLDER.

B. BLALOCK/MB

MAY 8, 1969   FAMILY CARE SUPERVISORY CALL: JOHN WAS IN SCHOOL BUT MRS. DELPH GAVE WORKER A COPY OF JOHN'S MOST RECENT REPORT CARD, DATED 4/25/69. JOHN RECEIVED FOUR "B'S" AND ONE "A". THE "A" WAS IN JOHN'S JOB TRAINING COURSE AND THE "B'S" WERE IN ENGLISH, MATH, SCIENCE AND PHYSICAL EDUCATION, SPECIAL EDUCATION COURSES. THE WORKER AND MRS. DELPH HAD A LONG DISCUSSION AS TO JOHN'S CONTINUED EXPRESSIONS TO THE FAMILY CARE PARENTS THAT PERHAPS HE WILL GO TO COLLEGE OR BE A PROFESSIONAL BALL PLAYER OF SOME SORT. THE WORKER INDICATED TO MRS. DELPH THAT IT WAS TIME WE STARTED BRINGING JOHN DOWN TO EARTH IN A SENSE THAT JOHN SHOULD REALIZE THAT IT TAKES A GREAT DEAL OF ABILITY TO BE ABLE TO GO TO COLLEGE AND THAT IT IS VERY DOUBTFUL THAT HE WOULD BE ABLE TO COLLEGE ENTRANCE EXAMINATIONS. I INDICATED TO MRS. DELPH THAT WE SHOULD TALK WITH JOHN ABOUT THIS, BIT WE SHOULD TALK TO HIM IN TERMS OF WHAT KIND OF JOB HE THINKS HE WILL LIKE BEST AND THAT HE SHOULD BE THINKING ABOUT THIS WHEN HE IS PLACED ON VARIOUS JOBS THROUGH THE JACKSON HIGH SCHOOL SPECIAL EDUCATION VOCATIONAL TRAINING COURSE. WE DISCUSSED WHAT SPECIAL EDUCATION CLASSES ARE AND THE FACT THAT HE IS RECEIVING MUCH OF THE SAME MATERIAL THAT REGULAR HIGH SCHOOL CHILDREN RECEIVE BUT THAT THE MATERIAL IS NOT PRESENTED TO HIM AS FAST AS IT IS TO

THE OTHER CHILDREN BECAUSE JOHN WOULD NOT BE ABLE TO LEARN AS MUCH IF IT WAS. A COPY OF JOHN'S REPORT CARD, DATED 4/25/69 IS FILED IN HIS FOLDER.

B. BLALOCK/A

JULY 8, 1969   JOHN IS EMPLOYED IN THE SUMMER RECREATION PROGRAM AS AN AIDE TO THE TEACHERS, AS IS INDICATED ABOVE. MR. SERGEANT IS JOHN'S IMMEDIATE SUPERVISOR AND IS A 6TH GRADE TEACHER DURING THE REGULAR SCHOOL SESSION. MR. SERGEANT IS VERY IMPRESSED WITH JOHN, KNOWING THAT JOHN IS FROM THIS INSTITUTION AND IS DIAGNOSED AS RETARDED…

B. BLALOCK/MB

JULY 16, 1969   F.C. SUPERVISORY CALL: JOHN WAS NOT HOME AT THE TIME OF THIS, CALL BUT MRS. DELPH INDICATED THAT SHE WOULD REMIND JOHN ABOUT SETTING A TIME TO VISIT HIS BROTHER IS HE SO WISHED SINCE IT WILL NOT BE LONG BEFORE SCHOOL WILL BE STATING. FILED IN JOHN'S FOLDER IS A POEM WROTE AND GAVE THE WORKER A COPY OF ENTITLED "HOW FAR MY LOVE". REFER TO IT FILED IN THE FOLDER DATED 6/16/69. JOHN ALSO GAVE THE WORKER ON 6/13/69 A COPY OF THE "SPORTS HIGHLIGHTS" THAT HE WROTE FOR THE SCHOOL PAPER. THESE WRITINGS INDICATE, I THINK, JOHN'S OUTGOING PERSONALITY AND GOOD EGO STRENGTH.

R. BLALOCK/MB

DEC. 2, 1969   F.C. TELEPHONE CALL FROM MISS GOLIAN, JOHN'S GRADE COUNSELOR AT JACKSON HIGH SCHOOL. SHE INDICATED THAT SHE HAS TALKED WITH THE SCHOOL'S WORK PLACEMENT COORDINATOR, A MR. HERENDEEN, AND THAT HE FEELS JOHN IS MAKING GOOD PROGRESS IN

SCHOOL, BUT HE WILL WORK WITH JOHN NEXT FALL EITHER THROUGH THE SPECIAL EDUCATION WORK EXPERIENCE PROGRAM OF THROUGH THE REGULAR CO-OP WORK PROGRAM.

R. BLALOCK/MB

SEPT. 18, 1969   JOHN IS PLAYING ON THE SCHOOL'S REGULAR FOOTBALL TEAM.

R. BLALOCK/EA

NOV. 20, 1969   FAMILY CARE COLLATERAL INTERVIEW: WORKER HAD AN INTERVIEW WITH JOHN'S GRADE COUNSELOR AT JACKSON HIGH SCHOOL, MISS GOOLIAN. SHE INDICATED THAT JOHN IS NOT REALISTIC IN THINKING OF FUTURE PLANS FOR HIMSELF AND THAT HE IS CURRENTLY TAKING DRAMATICS, BROADCASTING, ALONG WITH SOCIAL PROBLEMS, AMERICAN HISTORY AND ENGLISH. SHE SAID JOHN WILL NOT LISTEN TO HER IN A REASONING MANNER IF HE HAS AN IDEA IN HIS MIND. WE AGREED THAT WE HAVE TO GET JOHN PINNED DOWN TO REALITY SOON AND GUIDE HIM TOWARDS TAKING VOCATIONAL ORIENTED COURSES NEXT SEMESTER OR AT LEAST BY NEXT FALL. MISS GOOLIAN AGREED TO CONTACT THE SPECIAL EDUCATION WORK PLACEMENT COORDINATOR FOR THE HIGH SCHOOL AS TO THIS POSSIBLE CO-OP JOB ASSIGNMENT, AT LEAST BY NEXT FALL TERM – JOHN'S SENIOR YEAR. MISS GOOLIAN GAVE THE WORKER BRIEF WRITTEN REPORTS FROM JOHN'S FIVE TEACHERS. THESE REPORTS WERE ALL GLOWING REPORTS OF JOHN'S GOOD ATTITUDE TOWARD SCHOOL A INDICATED JOHN IS DOING FINE ACADEMIC WORK IN THESE NON-SPECIAL EDUCATION COURSES THIS SEMESTER. REFER TO THE REPORTS DATED NOVEMBER 18, 1969, FILED IN JOHN'S FOLDER.

R. BLALOCK/EA

FEB. 5, 1969   FAMILY CARE SUPERVISORY CALL: JOHN CAME HOME FROM
SCHOOL WHILE I WAS THERE AS THE SCHOOL HAD NO CLASSES IN THE
AFTERNOON. JOHN IS NOW QUITE A HUSKY FELLOW BEING ABOUT 6'2"
AND 190 POUNDS. HE IS LETTING HIS HAIR GROW IN THE AFRO-
AMERICAN STYLE. HE WAS DRESSED NEATLY AND COVERSED EASLILY
WITH THE WORKER. HE GAVE THE WORKER A COPY OF HIS GRADE
REPORTS WHICH INDICATED THAT HE RECEIVED 3RD SEMESTER MARKS
OF THREE "B'S", TWO "A'S" AND ONE "C", HAVING A 3 POINT AVERAGE.
THE "C" WAS IN AMERICAN HISTORY AND THE TWO "A'S" WERE IN
SOCIAL PROBLEMS AND PHYSICAL EDUCATION. REFER TO THE REPORTS
FILED IN JOHN'S FOLDER. JOHN GAVE THE WORKER A COPY OF A
SIMULATED LETTER HE HAD MADE UP ABOUT A SOLDIER IN VIET NAM.
HE SAID HE SENT PRESIDENT NIXON A COPY OF THIS LETTER AND
SHOWED THE WORKER A REPLY THAT HE HAD GOTTEN BACK THAT HE
GOTTEN BACK FROM THE WHITE HOUSE SECRETARY. BEFORE JOHN'S
ARRIVAL, WORKER DISCUSSED JOHN'S INDEPENDENT ATTITUDE AND
MATURING WITH MRS. DELPH. FOR EXAMPLE, HE WON'T PROBABLY
DISCUSS EVERY LITTLE THING WITH MR. AND MRS. DELPH AS HE HAS IN
THE PAST, SINCE HE IS NOW IN A STAGE WHERE HE WANT TO EXCERPT HIS
INDEPENDENCE AND PRIVACY MEANS A GREAT DEAL TO A TEENAGER.
R. BLALOCK/SK

JUNE 11, 1970   …WORKER ASKED JOHN ABOUT THIS FUTURE PLANS AFTER HIGH
SCHOOL AND HE TALKED A BIT MORE REALISTIC IN A SENSE THAT HE
MAY BE ABLE TO CONTINUE WORKING AT CONSUMER POWER COMPANY
OR HE MAY BE ELIGIBLE FOR SOME CLASSES AT JACKSON JUNIOR
COLLEGE. JOHN SAID HE WOULD LIKE TO BE AN AUTHOR SOMEDAY AND

HE SHOWED THE WORKER A BOOKLET HE HAD PREPARED OF THE POEMS HE HAS WRITTEN AS WELL AS SOME ARTICLES FOR THE SCHOOL PAPER. WE DISCUSSED QUALIFICATIONS FOR COLLEGE AND WHETHER OR NOT HE MAY BE ABLE TO ENTER. WE ALSO DISCUSSED THE COST INVOLVED IN FURTHER SCHOOLING AND THAT HE SHOULD SERIOUSLY CONSIDER COURSES NEXT YEAR WHICH MAY POINT HIM TOWARDS A VOCATIONAL TRAINING OR JOB ORIENTED CLASSES SINCE HE IS GOING TO HAVE TO WORK WHETHER OR NOT HE GOES TO COLLEGE. I RECOMMENDED HIM DISCUSSING IT FURTHER FOR MORE CLARIFICATION AS TO THE EXACT REQUIREMENTS, WITH HIS SCHOOL GRADE COUNSELOR, MISS GOOLIAN. JOHN TOOK THE DRAMATICS COURSE AT THE SCHOOL AND WAS REPORTEDLY IN THE SCHOOL PLAY. HE AMITTED THAT HE DID NOT KNOW OR UNDERSTATND MUCH OF THE PLAY WHICH APPARENTLY WAS A SHAKESPEAREAN PLAY. R. BLALOCK/SK

JUNE 11, 1970   OUTPATIENT NOTE: WORKER LATER SPOKE ON THE TELEPHONE WITH JOHN'S GRADE COUNSELOR, MISS GOOLIAN. SHE INDICATED THAT SHE HAS SPOKEN AT SOME LENGTH WITH JOHN ABOUT THE SUBJECT HE HAS TAKEN IN SCHOOL AND THAT IN HER OPINION, HE IS NOT TAKING JOB ORIENTING OR VOCATIONAL ORIENTING COURSES. SHE INDICATED THAT JOHN DROPPED A GEOGRAPHY CLASS THIS PAST SPRING BECAUSE HE WAS NOT DOING WELL IN IN AND BECAUSE HE WANTED TO KEEP A 3 POINT GRADE AVERAGE, WHICH HE NOW HAS. HOWEVER, SHE SAID THE 3 POINT GRADE AVERAGE DOES NOT MEAN A THING IF JOHN CONTINUES TO TAKE THE SIMPLE COURSES WHICH DO NOT PREPARE HIM FOR COPING WITH JOB SITUATIONS WHEN SCHOOL IS NO LONGER AVAILABLE FOR JOHN. MISS GOOLIAN INDICATED THAT SHE HAD TALKED WITH THE SPECIAL EDUCATIONAL VOCATIONAL PLACEMENT COORDINATOR AND THAT HE

INDICATED TO HER THAT HE DID NOT FEEL JOHN SHOULD BE IN HIS PROGRAM SINCE JOHN WAS ALREADY DEMONSTRATING SOCIALLY ACCEPTABLE BEHAVIOR AND CAPABLE OF MANY MORE THINGS THAN THE STUDENTS HE NOW SERVES. A SPECIAL EDUCATION TEACHER THAT HAS HAD JOHN IN HER CLASSES LAST YEAR ALSO INDICATED THAT SHE DID NOT FEEL JOHN SHOULD BE IN THESE SPECIAL EDUCATIONAL VOCATIONAL PLACEMENT PROGRAMS. JOHN HAS HAD REGULAR CLASS THIS YEAR BUT THREE OF THESE HAVE BEEN RELATIVELY EASY CLASSES. THESE ARE DRAMATICS, BROADCASTING AND PHYSICAL EDUCATION. MISS GOOLIAN INDICATED THAT THE SCHOOL HAD SELECTED JOHN, ALONG WITH 17 OTHER STUDENTS IN THE 11TH GRADE TO WORK AT CONSUMER POWER COMPANY ON VARIOUS JOBS, SUCH AS TRANSPORTING MATERIALS AND, TRANSFERRING FIGURES FROM ONE PLACE TO ANOTHER OR ONE COLUMN TO ANOTHER. JOHN WILL REPORTEDLY WORK FIVE DAYS A WEEK, 40 HOURS PER WEEK BEGINNING JUNE 15TH TO SEPTEMBER 4TH, EARNING $1.60 PER HOUR. WORKER DISCUSSED BRIEFLY JOHN'S IDEA THAT HE CAN GO TO COLLEGE BECAUSE OF HIS 3 POINT GRADE AVERAGE. SHE FEELS THIS WOULD NOT BE GOOD FOR JOHN TO ENTER INTO A COLLEGE PROGRAM IF HE COULD FIND FINANCIAL HELP WHICH SHE FEELS HE MIGHT BE ABLE TO DO THROUGH THE MARTIN LUTHER KING SCHOLARSHIP FUND, BECAUSE HE WOULD NOT BE READY FOR SUCH AN ACADEMIC PROGRAM SINCE HE CAN NOT DO GOOD ACADEMIC WORK IN HIGH SCHOOL. WORKER INDICATED TO MISS GOOLIAN THAT I WOULD TALK WITH JOHN MORE THIS FALL IN REGARD TO JOHN AND THE POSSIBLE COURSES HE MAY BE ABLE TO TAKE WHICH MIGHT PREPARE HIM BETTER FOR A JOB AFTER SCHOOL. HOWEVER, JOHN HAS APPARENTLLY SIGNED UP FOR COURSES NEXT FALL.

R. BLALOCK/SK

AUG. 25, 1970

FAMILY CARE SUPERVISORY CALL: ON 8/20/70, WORKER SAW MR. AND MRS. DELPH AT THEIR HOME. MR. DELPH WAS ON VACATION. WE DISCUSSED IN SOME DETAIL JOHN'S SOMEWHAT UNREALISTIC ATTITUDE IN THE PAST ABOUT GOING TO COLLEGE OR PLAYING PROFESSIONAL FOOTBALL AFTER HIGH SCHOOL. THEY REALIZE IT SEEMS, TOO, THAT JOHN WILL NOT BE ABLE TO DO THESE THINGS; THAT WE ALL HAVE OUR LIMITATIONS BOTH PHYSICAL AND MENTAL. WE AGREED THAT WE SHOULD, WHENEVER POSSIBLE, BRING JOHN DOWN TO EARTH , SO TO SPEAK, BY TALKING WITH HIM ABOUT WHAT KIND OF JOBS HE MAY BE QUALIFIED FOR AND TO GET HIM TO THINKING IN TERMS OF WORKING AFTER HIGH SCHOOL OR PERHAPS TO TAKE A COURSE OR TWO IN A JUNIOR COLLEGE LEVEL. WORKER POINTED OUT THAT THE REAL POSSIBLE EMOTIONAL FRUSTRATION THAT COULD BE INVOLVED IF JOHN WAS BY CHANCE ACCEPTED INTO A COLLEGE AND JUST COULD NOT DO THE REQUIRED ACADEMIC MATERIAL, AS IT SEEMS HE WILL NOT BE ABLE TO DO, SINCE HE IS TESTING IN THE HANDICAPPED..... MR. DELPH SEEMS TO BE ABLE TO BE FIRM WITH JOHN IN APPROPRIATE SITUATIONS AND YET FAIR AT THE SAME TIME. HE INDICATED THAT JOHN HAD WANTED TO QUIT HIS JOB IN ORDER TO PRACTICE FOOTBALL, BUT MR. DELPH POINTED OUT TO JOHN THAT THIS JOB WOULD ONLY LAST WEEK OR SO AND THIS WEEK COULD VERY WELL BE IMPORTANT TO HIS FUTURE IN TERMS OF GETTING THAT JOB AFTER SCHOOL; WHEREAS PLAYING FOOTBALL IS IMPORTANT TOO, BUT THIS IS SOMETHING HE WILL NOT BE ABLE TO DO ON A TEAM LEVEL AFTER HIGH SCHOOL, AND THAT THEREFORE, THE JOB IS VERY IMPORTANT.

R. BLALOCK/SLH

OCT. 9, 1970   FAMILY CARE SUPERVISORY CALLS: JOHN HAS BEEN AGAIN QUALIFIED TO PLAY ON THE VARSITY FOOTBALL TEAM AT JACKSON AS MRS. DELPH INDICATED THAT HE IS PRACTICING EVERY NIGHT EXCEPT THE WEEKENDS AND SEEMS TO ENJOY IT VERY MUCH. JOHN IS APPARENTLY A SCHOOL NEWSPAPER STAFF MEMBER AND AS PART OF HIS JOB IS TO REPORT AND WRITE UP INFORMATION AS TO THE SCHOOL SPORT ACTIVITIES AND RESULTS. WORKER DISCUSSED BRIEFLY WITH MRS. DELPH WHETHER JOHN'S ATTITUDE TOWARDS A JOB OPPORTUNITY AT SCHOOL HAS CHANGED AND SHE INDICATED THAT JOHN TALKS A GREAT DEAL NOW ABOUT BEING A NEWS OR SPORTS ANNOUNCER FOR JACKSON HIGH SCHOOL. WORKER INDICATED THAT I WOULD BE SEEING JOHN AND HIS SCHOOL COUNSELOR IN THE NEAR FUTURE TO HELP TRY TO COORDINATE SOME OF JOHN'S PLANS INTO REALISTIC CHANNELS FOR HIM.

R. BLALOCK/SH

NOV. 21, 1970   WORK SPOKE WITH JOHN'S SCHOOL COUNSELOR, MR. HUBERT FURNACE, WHO INDICATED THAT HE WILL WRITE TO WESTERN MICHIGAN UNIVERSITY, AS JOHN REQUESTED, FOR A POSSIBLE SCHOLARSHIP FOR JOHN. MR. FURNACE EXPLAINED THAT WESTERN HAS A SPECIFIC PROGRAM FOR DISADVANTAGED MINORITY GROUP YOUTH WHO WILL BE GRADUATING FROM HIGH SCHOOL. ACCORDING TO MR. FURNACE, WESTERN MICHIGAN UNIVERSITY WOULD COUNSEL JOHN THROUGHOUT THE FIRST YEAR OR TWO, AS WELL AS PROVIDE EMPLOYMENT ON THE GROUNDS FOR HIM TO HELP PAY TOWARDS THE COST OF HIS ROOM AND PROVIDE BOARD. JOHN WAS BROUGHT INTO THE DISCUSSION AT THIS TIME AND INDICATED HIS DESIRE TO PROCEED WITH THAT PROGRAM IF AT ALL POSSIBLE.

DEC. 2, 1970   WORKER SPOKE WITH MR, AND MRS. DELPH IN REGARD TO JOHN'S PLAN TO ENTER COLLEGE. WORKER ASKED THEM IF THEY WOULD BE WILLING TO GIVE JOHN ROOM AND BOARD IF JOHN IS PLACED ON CONVALESCENT STATUS DURING THE TIME HE ENTERS COLLEGE. WORKER INDICATED THAT, ACCORDING TO MR. FURNACE, JOHN'S COUNSELOR, JOHN WOULD SPEND MUCH OR MOST OF HIS TIME AT THE SCHOOL IF HE IS ACCEPTED, BUT THAT JOHN FEELS AND THINKS OF THE DELPHS AS HIS HOME. MR. AND MRS. DELPH SAID AS FAR AS THEY WERE CONCERNED, THIS IS JOHN'S HOMES AND THEY WOULD LET HIM STAY WITH THEM WHILE HE WAS GOING TO COLLEGE, EVEN THOUGH HE WOULD BE UNABLE TO PAY FOR ROOM AND BOARD.

APRIL 22, 1971   FAMILY CARE SUPERVISORY CALLS AND NOTE: MRS. DELPH AGAIN INDICATED THAT THEY WOULD CONTINUE TO CARE FOR JOHN AS THEY THOUGHT OF HIM NOW AS PART OF THEIR FAMILY. MRS. DELPH GAVE THE WORKER A COPY OF JOHN'S ACADEMIC ATTENDANCE AND CITIZENSHIP REPORT FROM JACKSON HIGH SCHOOL DATED 3/21/71. THE SCHOOL REPORT INDICATED THAT JOHN IS RECEIVING "A'S" AND "B'S". MRS. DELPH ALSO GAVE THE WORKER A COPY OF THE SCHOOL BULLETIN CALLED THE "VIKING TRACK", OF WHICH JOHN WRITES ABOUT THE SPORTS PROGRAM. JOHN IS PARTICIPATING IN THE JACKSON HIGH SCHOOL TRACK PROGRAM AND HE IS RUNNING IN THE 440 YARD DASH AS WELL AS THE 220 YARD DASH. HE CONTINUES TO BE ACTIVE IN THE SCHOOL PROGRAMS SUCH AS BROADCASTING, DRAMATICS CLUB AND THE SCHOOL AND CHURCH CHOIRS.

B. BLALOCK/SH

JUNE 6, 1971   FAMILY CARE NOTE; WORKER TELEPHONED THE KENT COUNTY PROBATE COURT, REGISTRAR'S OFFICE, AND TALKED WITH A MRS.

CHASES, DEPUTY REGISTRAR. MRS. CHASES INDICATED THAT THE KENT COUNTY PROBATE COURT WOULD ACCEPT A PETITION FROM JOHN AFTER HE HAS BEEN DISCHARGED FROM THE INSTITUTION ONE YEAR OR LONGER FOR A RESTORATION OF RIGHTS WITHOUT THE NEED OF DOCTORS REPORTS RECOMMENDING THE SAME. MRS. CHASES INDICATED THAT SINCE IN OUR OPINION, JOHN WAS NOT IN NEED OF A LEGAL OR GUARDIAN OF AN ESTATE, THAT THERE WOULD BE NO PROBLEMS WITH HIS PLNS TO ENTER COLLEGE OR BE ON HIS OWN.

R. BLALOCK/SH

MAY 25, 1971   WORKER CALLED MR. HUBERT FURNACE, JACKSON HIGH SCHOOL COUNSELOR FOR JOHN. MR. FURNACE INDICATED THAT JOHN HAD BEEN ACCEPTED DEFINITELY INTO THE MARTIN LUTHER KING SCHOLARSHIP PROGRAM FOR ADMISSION TO WESTERN MICHIGAN UNIVERSITY AND THAT JOHN WILL BE PARTICIPATING IN AN ORIENTATION PROGRAM AND DEVELOPMENT FOR ATTITUDES PROGRAM FROM JUNE 21 TO SOMETIME IN AUGUST. MR. FURNACE INDICATED THAT JOHN WOULD BE RESIDING AT THE SCHOOL IN DORMITORIES WITH OTHER STUDENTS IN THAT PROGRAM AND THAT IN SEPTEMBER THEY WOULD BE BACK AT THE UNIVERSITY FOR REGULAR SCHOOL CLASSES.

R. BLALOCK/SH

JUNE 17, 1971   FAMILY CARE SUPERVISORY CALL: JOHN WAS HOME AND WAS VERY PROUD OF HIS HIGH SCHOOL DIPLOMA HE RECEIVED LAST EVENING, 6/16/71, AS WELL AS THE FACT THAT HE GRADUATED WITH SCHOLASTIC HONORS HAVING A 3.0 GRADE AVERAGE FOR HIS HIGH SCHOOL YEARS. WORKER SPOKE AT LENGTH, WITH JOHN IN REGARD TO THE FACT THAT SINCE HE IS NOW GRADUATING FROM HIGH SCHOOL AND WILL BE ENTERING COLLEGE STUDY THIS SUMMER, THAT THE STAFF AT THE

INSTITUTION INCLUDING MYSELF, WOULD RECOMMEND THAT HE BE DISCHARGED FROM THE JURISDICTION OF CSH&TS. THIS APPARENTLY WAS A LITTLE FRIGHTENING FOR JOHN TO ACCEPT ALTHOUGH HE WAS REASSURED THAT HE CAN STILL CONTACT US AND ALSO THAT HE COULD CONTACT THE JACKSON HIGH SCHOOL COUNSELORS FOR ASSISTANCE IN PROBLEMS HE MAY IN THE FUTURE. JOHN WAS ENTHUSIASTIC ABOUT ENTERING THE SUMMER SCHOOL PROGRAM AT WESTERN AND SHOWED THE WORKER THE $2,000 GRANT HE RECEIVED FOR THE FALL TERM AND THE GRANT HE RECEIVED FOR THE SEVEN WEEK SUMMER PROGRAM. WORKER DOES NOT FEEL JOHN WOULD HAVE VERY MANY PROBLEMS IN FINDING A JOB, IN FACT, HE IS EXCLUDED FROM THE UNIVERSITY PROGRAM THIS SUMMER OR FALL. JOHN'S EFFERESCENT PERSONALITY AND ABILITY TO MEET AND TALK WITH PEOPLE WILL ENABLE HIM TO USE HIS SOCIAL HABITS WHICH ARE VERY GOOD IN THAT HE DOES NOT APPEAR TO WANT TO DRINK OR SMOKE EXCESSIVELY NOR ASSOCIATE WITH PEOPLE WHO WOULD WANT TO EXPLOIT HIM.

JULY 14, 1971   FAMILY CARE NOTE: FILED IN JOHN'S FOLDER IS A LETTER FROM HIS FAMILY CARE PARENTS BEFORE HE WAS DISCHARGED INDICATING THEIR INTENTION OF OFFERING A HOME FOR JOHN AS LONG AS HE WISHES TO STAY WITH THEM.

R. BLALOCK/PL

JULY 9, 1971   DISCHARGED FROM THE INSTITUTION EFFECTIVE UNDER SECTION 25A, PUBLIC ACT 151 OF 923, AS AMENDED BY PUBLIC ACT OF 1937. KENT COUNTY PROBATE COURT NOTIFIED.

DISCHARGE SUMMARY ATTACHED.

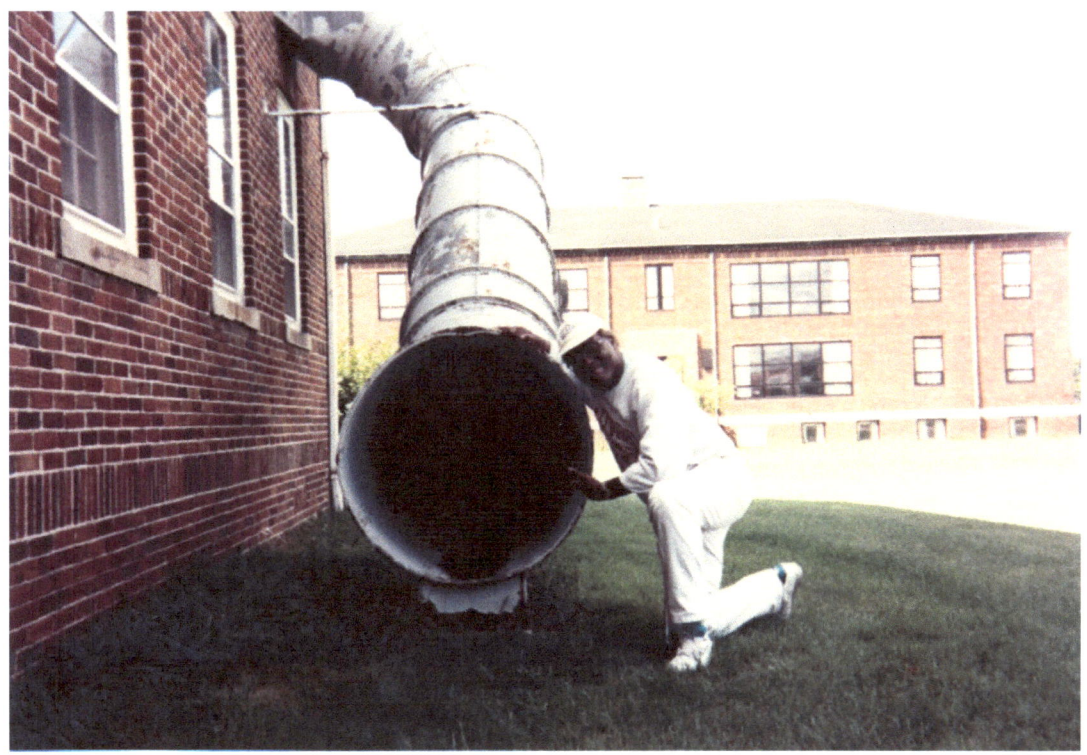

Above and Below: This is the fire escape at the institution where I once hid to avoid an

overweight supervisor

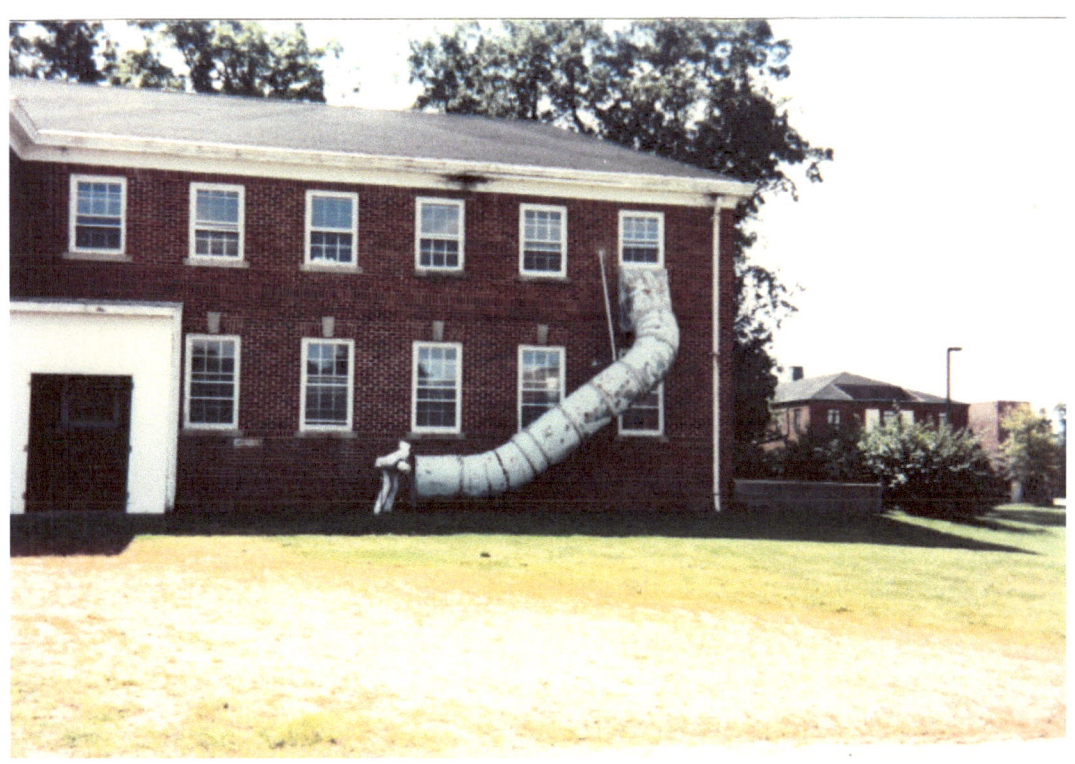

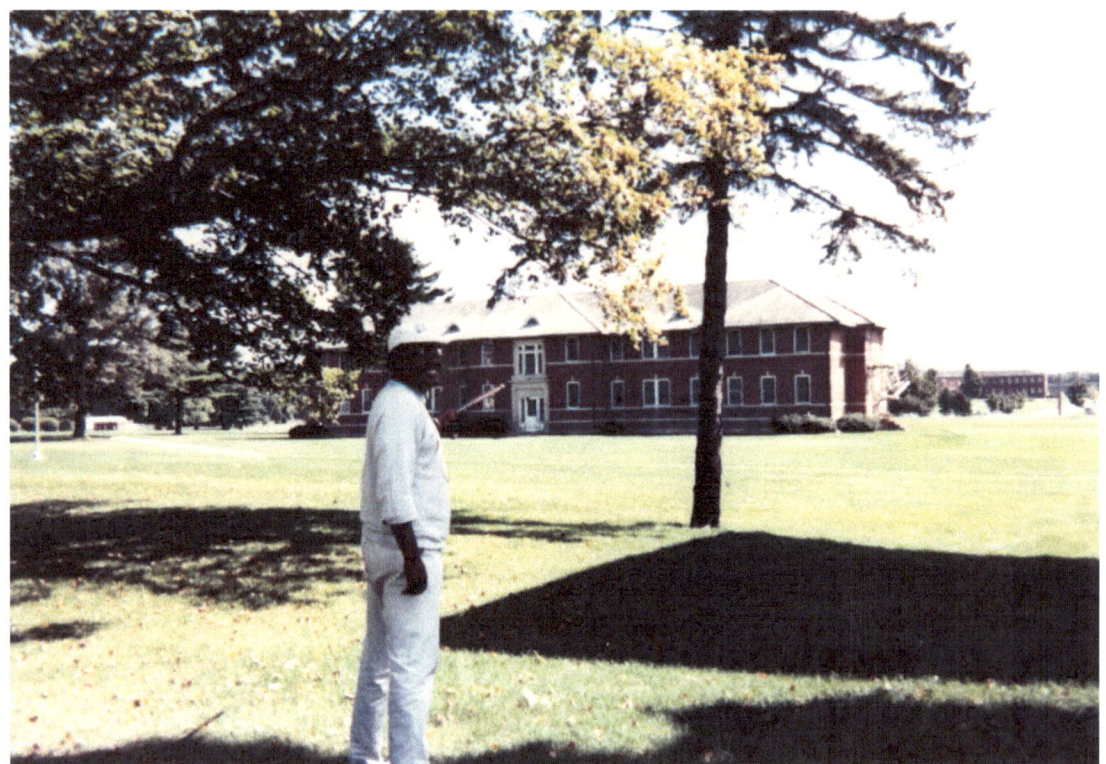

One of the Few Woman housing units

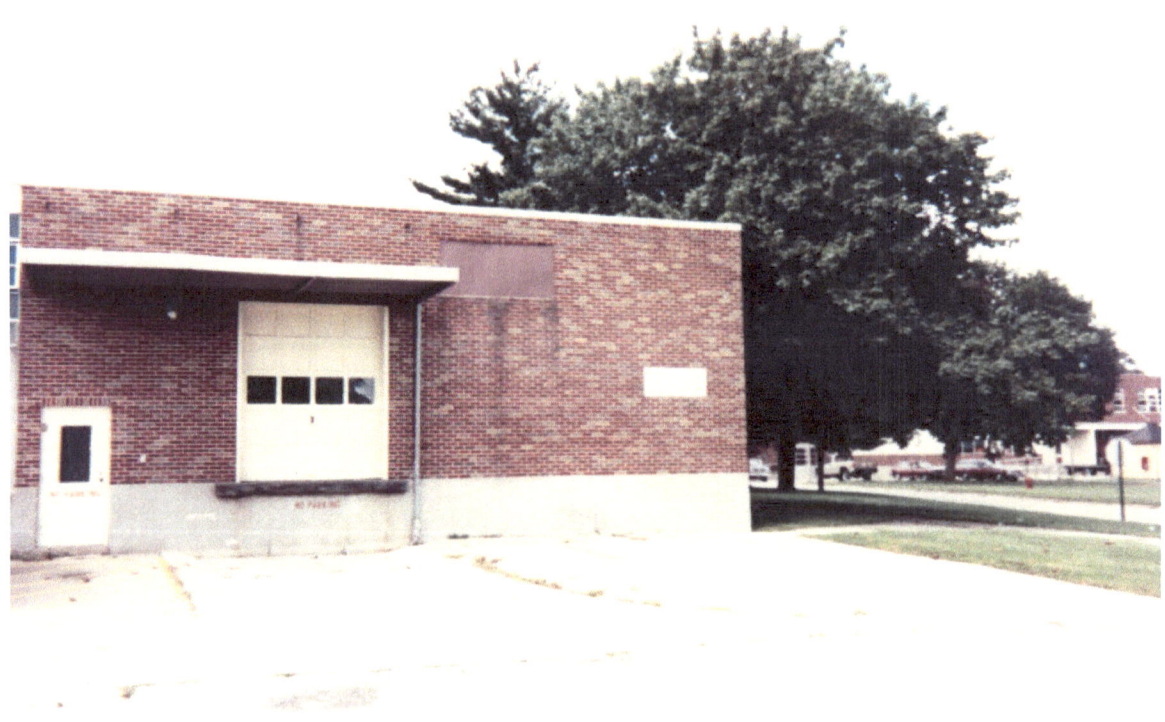

The laundry room on the grounds of the institution

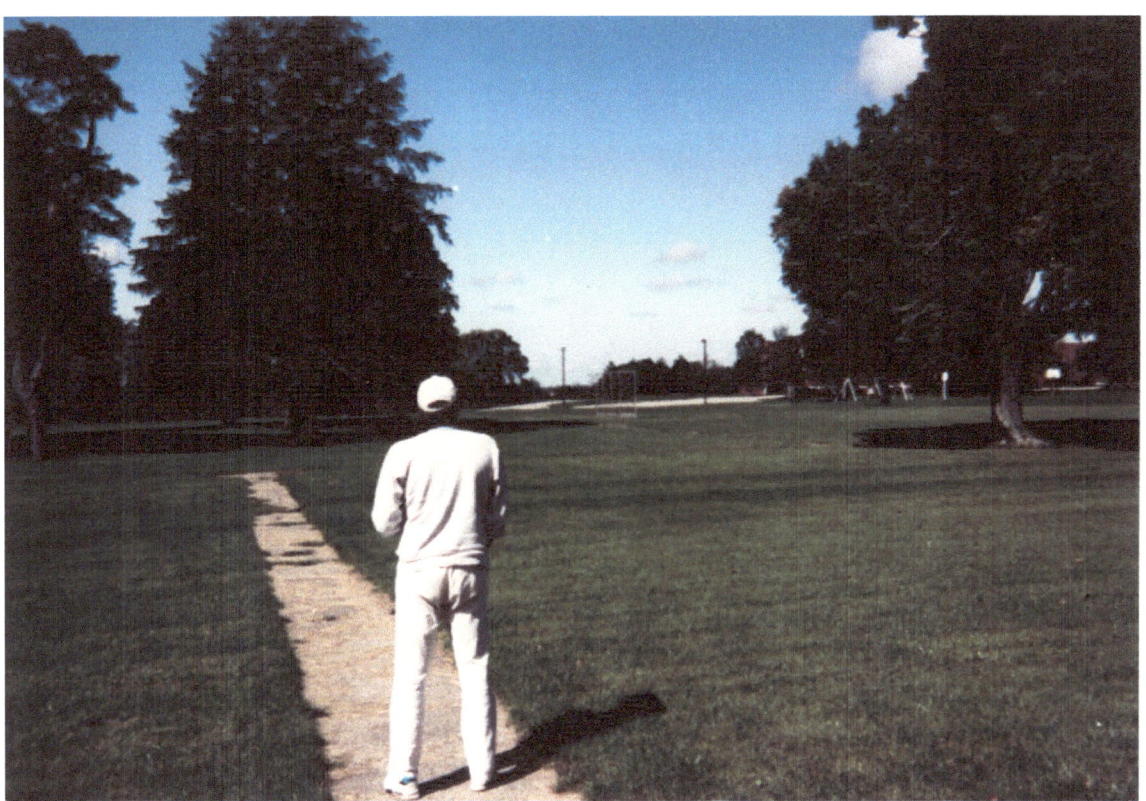

The long walk to chow hall

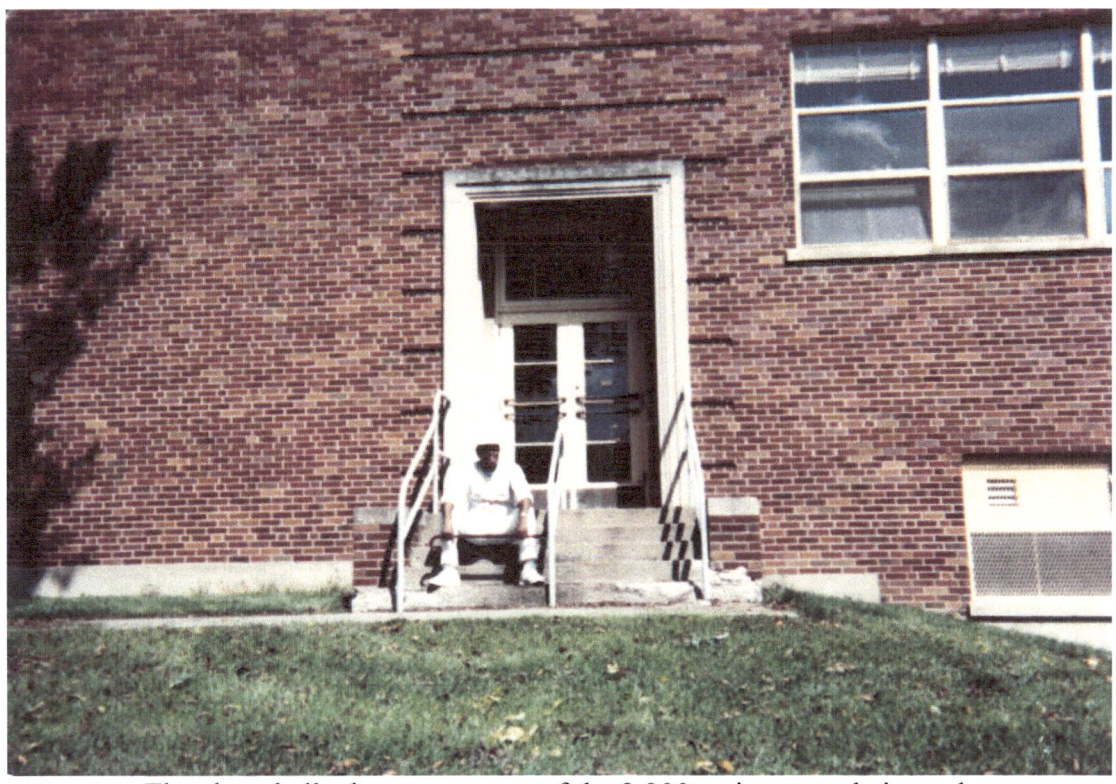

The chow hall where every one of the 2,900 patients ate their meals

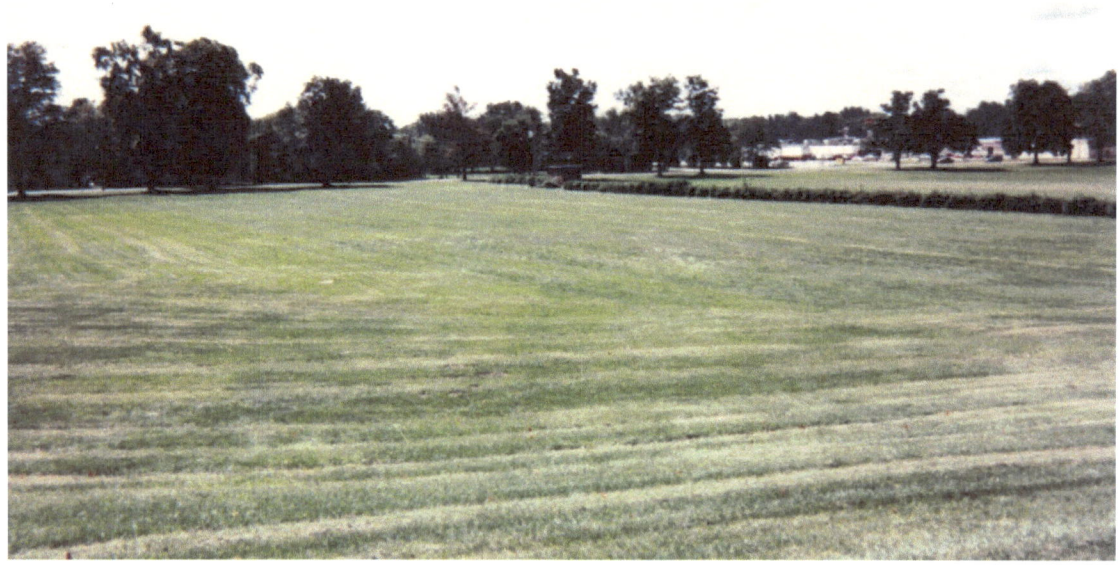

The open field where we played sports. If you look closely you will see a long line of brushes where I fell into a hornets nest. I became a track star at that moment

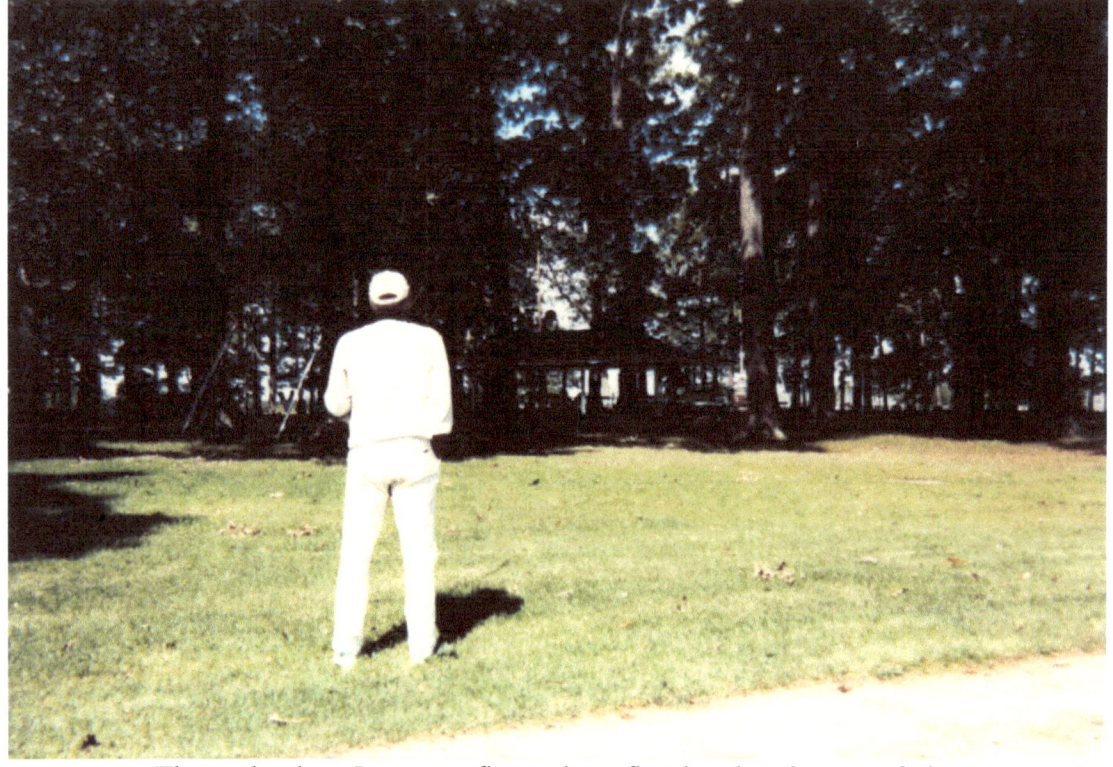

The park where I saw my first twister first hand at the age of nine

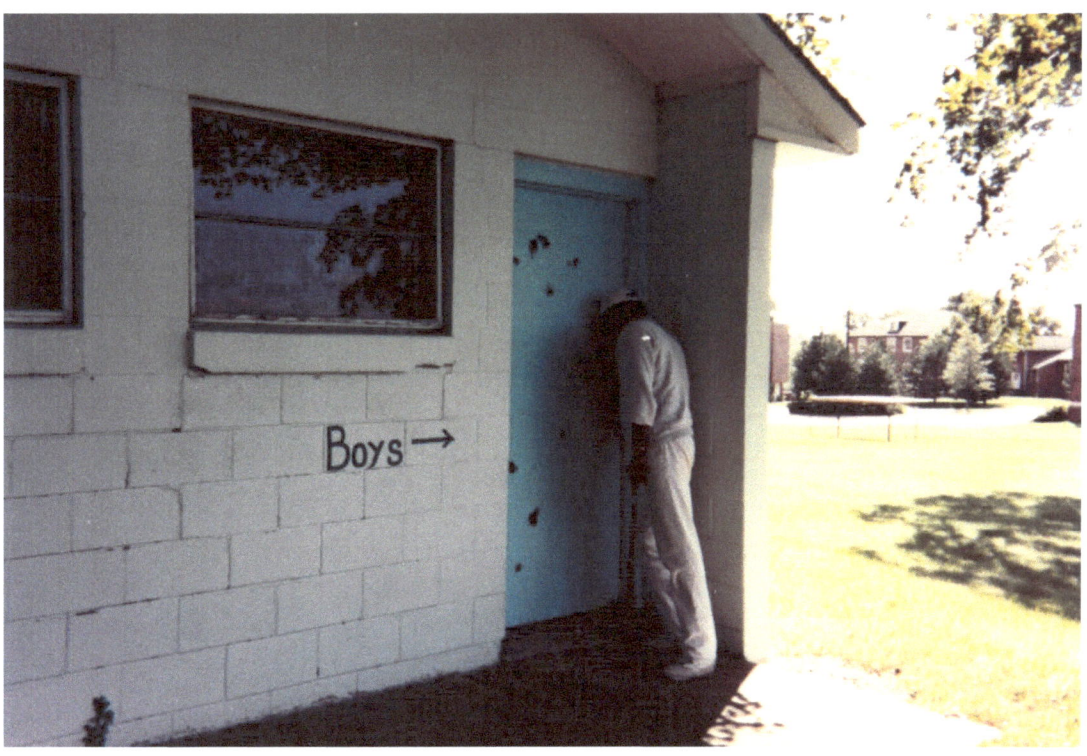

Above and Below: This is me sneaking a peek into the Boy's restroom across from the housing unit I lived in

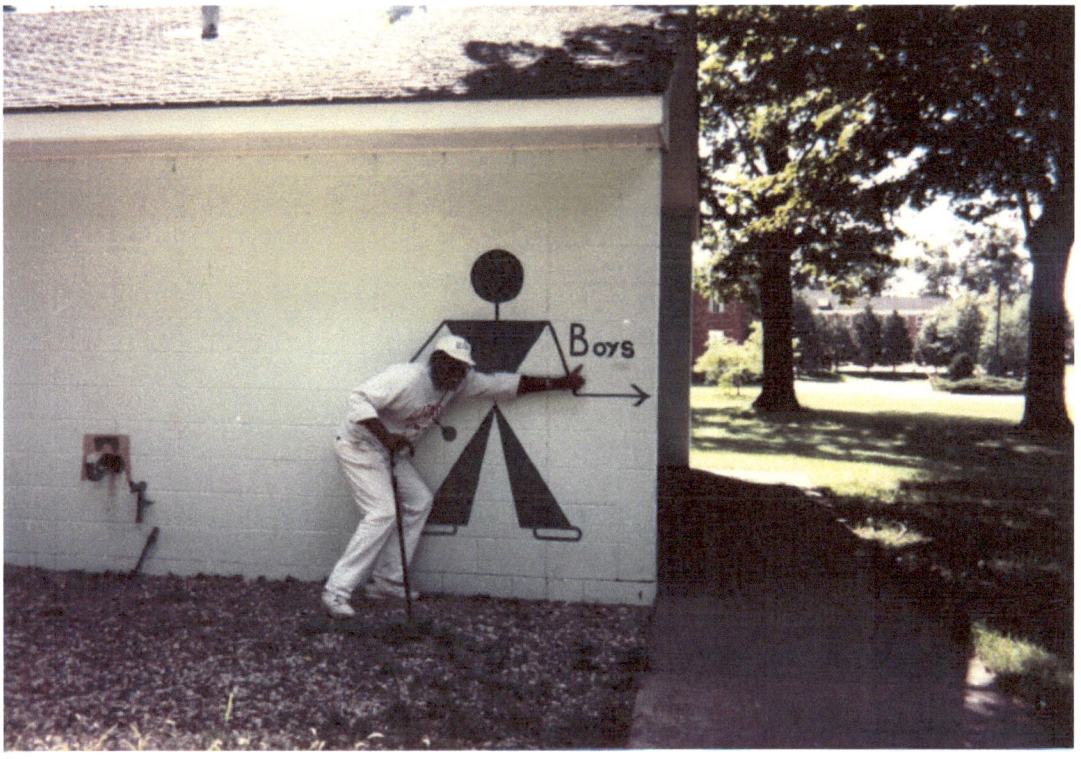

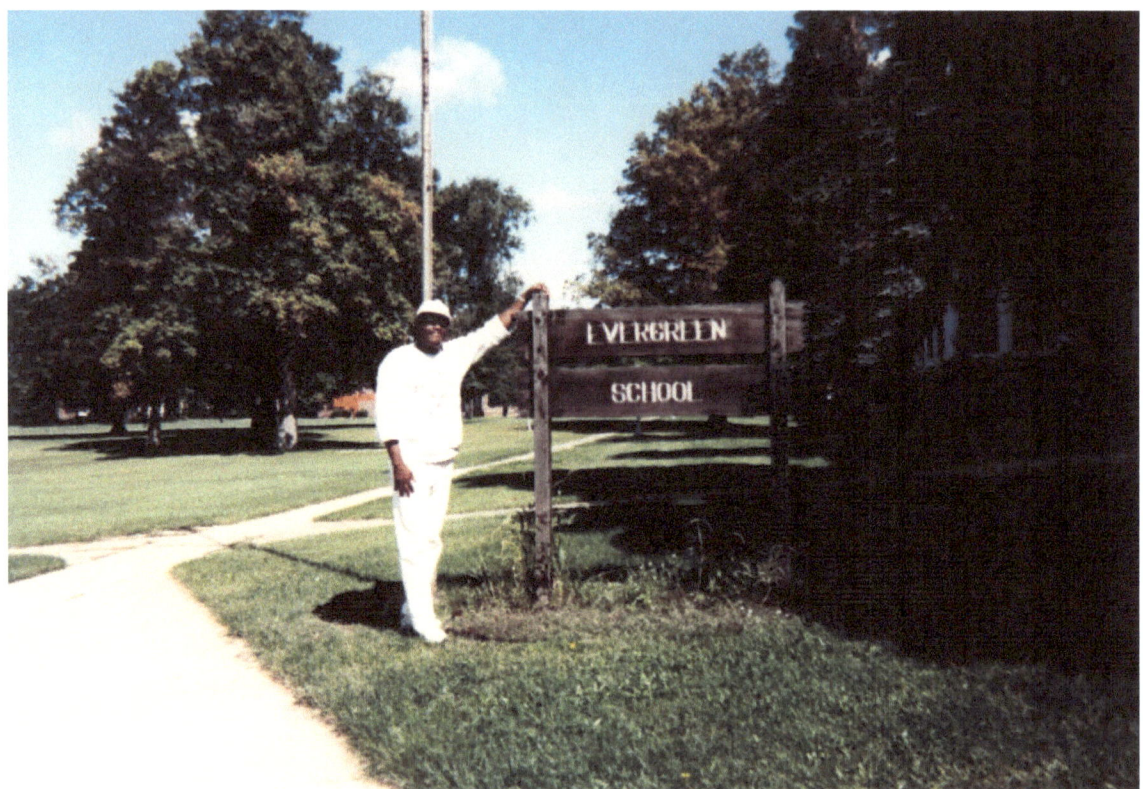

Full circle! Evergreen School at the Institution now a Prison. I once taught there!

Left To Do It Alone

The Author

Refusing to accept derogatory titles attached to him by society and determined to make it in an often unfriendly world, John Pharms, a ward of the courts at the age of eight months, stands today as testimony to the virtue of self-determination.

The 6'3" 240 pound former athlete, who is today a vocational education teacher at the Latham School in Brewster, Massachusetts on Cape Cod, has come a long way from that day thirty seven years ago when he and his twin brother were taken away from their natural parents. John Pharms had to spend many years in institutions with mentally handicapped children, an unpromising start to life, one that might have depressed and finished many but not Pharms

After receiving his discharge papers upon graduating from high school, Pharms attended and graduated from Western Michigan University in Kalamazoo, Michigan. Pharms received a Thurgood Marshall Scholarship to attend graduate school after which he opted to return to his high school alma mater to teach and coach.

From high school coaching, Pharms moved on to coach on the collegiate level when he joined the football coaching staff at Lincoln Missouri University as defensive line coach. It was here that Pharms met Archie Moore, the former Light Heavyweight Boxing Champion of the world. Archie's son, Hardy, was a standout wide receiver for the Blue Tiger (school nickname) football team.

Then it was back to Mallorca, Spain, where Pharms had previously done his student teaching. This time, he was both athletic director and the head basketball coach. The high school's Fighting Eagles Basketball Team became one of the best in Spain under his leadership. While in Spain, Pharms also traveled with the Gold Medal World Junior (USA) Championship Basketball Team that featured the New York Knick's Kenny Walker of the National Basketball League.

After two years on Spain's beautiful Mediterranean Island, Pharms decided to make the move to Denmark, settling in the country's second largest city, Arhus. He had accepted the basketball coaching post of a local Division I professional league. Pharms returned to the States after the Chernobyl nuclear disaster and after terrorist attacks against Americans.

Pharms lived in Raleigh, North Carolina, where he was befriended by Billy Graham's son-in-law and was signed up to do a basketball camp with the late National Basketball Hall of Fame member, " Pistol" Pete Maravich.

Looking for rest, Pharms relocated to Cape Cod. Instead he found a job at the Latham School working with mentally retarded young adults. He has appeared in numerous plays as well as in a small character part on "Unsolved Mysteries" for national television.

Fed up with life? Down on you luck? Looking for an identity? After reading this book, I guarantee that you will want to redirect your energy to become the best that you can be. After all, isn't this what this story has proven? In this country, regardless of race, creed or color, anyone can succeed who is willing to work for it!

Read a book! Better, perhaps, finish this one and get a new start with your life.

Opening Anecdote

My closest friend in the Coldwater, Michigan Institution was a hydrocephalic boy whose name I have forgotten, but whose friendship I shall never forget. We used to say what when we got out of there, we were going to do such and such. My friend never made it. He was killed by another patient who made him eat floor wax and hit him on the head with a cast. Then my friend fell from the porch of the cottage on his head. I vowed at that moment that I would make it for the both of us.

Introduction

While a student in college, I attempted to sit down and write a book I felt would make good reading, considering that it would be about my life. For fifteen years, I have been telling myself that no one would want to read a story about an unknown. I felt such stories were reserved for star athletes, politicians, or the children of movie idols. I kept reassuring myself that there is room for a story about a 37 year old man who teaches mentally retarded people. Now you might ask, what is so unique about this? How about the fact that I spent twenty years being raised in a licensed boarding home, state institutions and foster homes? I felt that if anyone was going to write this story, it would have to be written by me.

You may ask, what is so unique about this story? There have been many stories about children born into more disadvantaged situations who have gone to achieve great things in life. What would warrant me the right to share such at story? A story of a drunken father and a promiscuous mother is commonplace today. This type of story headlines many of our newspapers every day. What can be said that hasn't already been said about the cruelty that has been inflicted upon our children by parents who were either too young to be such, or by parents who were abused themselves? This could be just another one of those stories. But I stand ready to argue that this is not just another one of those stories. Indeed, this is not about immigrant Europeans arriving on Ellis Island or emancipated slaves escaping via the Underground Railroad. This story is of a boy who was left to do it alone.

There are many children out there who have come through life without a father or a mother. These same children do not know what it's like to have parental support or an environment free of drugs and crime. These same children have had to battle for years an identity of not knowing who they really are. I remember telling my foster care family that I am not interested in changing my last name to theirs. I wanted to have something that I could identify as my own.

This is my opportunity to voice my concern for the unheard. My one opportunity to break the silent, but painful echoing of abused children's voices everywhere. My crusade is to reach these children either black or white. To inform them that excellence in athletics is not the quick road to the fast lane. That the road to success by way of athletic competition is a long one cluttered with broken promises, unfulfilled dreams to make the professional sports circuit, used up athletic scholarships, and the result: a young man or woman with faded memories, yet unemployed. Nothing is worse than to see a bright, inner city or suburban young person fall prey to greedy and unconcerned adults, and who later becomes unemployed in a society where he or she is no longer the hero. This story is dedicated to neglected and abused children everywhere. To me, they are the true heroes. My challenge is that you live life to the fullest.

This institution where I was placed was established in 1863 for the care of the mentally retarded. It was providing residential care for some 12,500 patients. Coldwater housed 2,900 patients of which 450 were being trained for jobs that would eventually take them out of the institution, while 175 children were being treated in the academic program. I was one of those students. My record now reflects a deed paid back to society.

The building and places in this story are real, but some of the names have been changed to protect the identity of those people who may still be living.

The Institutional Years

As I look back and reflect upon the institution where I was raised, it is very difficult for me to put into words all the things that happened there. After a short stay with my Aunt and Uncle in Grand Rapids, I was placed in the protective custody of the state courts at Fort Custer State Home and Training School. The year was 1956 and I was four years of age. The institution had just been reopened and welcomed 1,200 patients. The institution, known as the Percy Jones Hospital Annex, had been used as a base hospital for training during World War II. I don't remember too much about Fort Custer. I remember walking with my brother and sister one day, and the next, I was there.

One incident that I've never forgotten occurred when a boy from our building decided to run away. No one knew where he had gone, so they brought in a helicopter. I ran and hid, fearful that it would eat me. One of the supervisors reassured me that it was not a giant grasshopper, and I went out to join the search. I had never seen so many G-I Joe's in my life! "What a collection of tanks, jeeps, helicopters and soldiers", I thought to myself. It took them four hours, but they did manage to find him hiding underneath one of our buildings.

During the winter, we would take our sleds and go sledding down one of the hills in front of our building. When the weather was warm, we would go play Cowboys and Indians. In between, I was given a series of tests that diagnosed me as a high grade moron. Continued testing over the next few years still classified me as either a low or high grade moron.

While my twin brother and I were living in Fort Custer, we were befriended by a local worker by the name of Gradie Dawson who lived in Battle Creek. Gradie would often visit and take us on weekend visits to his family home. The visits continued even after we were transferred to Coldwater State Home and Training School in the winter of 1960.

The long drive from Battle Creek to Coldwater was very quiet as my twin brother, Jimmy, and I clung to each other in anticipation of yet another new place to adjust to. In eight years of life, we had five different places to call home.

Upon our arrival, we were assigned to Cottage 8 dormitory. We figured every kid in the world traveled and lived the way we did. We were introduced to the Cottage 8 residents and started questioning them when a huge man, Mr. Pringer, came out and hit my brother in the stomach with a billy club and promptly ordered, "We don't talk here unless you are told to do so, understand?" Jimmy started crying, and Mr. Pringer informed me that unless I made him stop, he would receive more of the same. I comforted my brother, and we sat ourselves down with the rest of the kids.

Two adult supervisors ran each dormitory in the institution. To the best of my recollection, there were five dormitories for men and also five for the women. There were buildings for athletics, meals, a hospital, and a jail-type dormitory for patients who ran away or were caught in the act of committing a crime. In this building, the residents' hair was shaved and they were fed bread and water. Very well hidden in the forest was another group of buildings that housed the physically impaired and the emotionally unstable.

There were two things we had to do our first day at the institution. We had to fight and wrestle the best kid in boxing and I lost to Joe, the best kid in wrestling. Joe was choking me to death, and Mr. Pringer was not about to stop him, so I promised to do anything for him if he would let me go. Later Joe and I became the best of friends during my stay at Coldwater.

I was transferred from Cottage 8 to Cottage 5 and away from Mr. Pringer. But Mr. Owens at Cottage 5 seemed to be a clone of Mr. Pringer. Mr. Owens would put a kid in the middle of a circle and have all the kids jump on top of him until he was satisfied. I was one was put in the sick game. I remember almost suffocating to death. An intriguing thing Mr. Owens did occurred one day when another kid and I were arguing, and this kid called me "a nigger". When I informed Mr. Owens of this incident, he took this kid inside, punished him and brought him back outside and made him apologize to me. Mr. Owens told this kid that he was no better than me. A strange revelation considering this was 1962, and the Civil Rights Bill would not be passed until 1964. Hearing this from a white man made me realize that I could do anything I wanted if I was willing to work hard for it.

It was during this period as a student that word came to our class about President John F. Kennedy being killed by a sniper. After this major event I was transferred from Cottage 5 to Cottage 1, which was one step away from being placed in foster care. By this time, Gradie Dawson had stopped seeing us for reasons unknown, but we were being considered for foster care placement as soon as suitable families could be located.

Life up to that point seemed to be one struggle after another for me: pneumonia and meningitis at eight months, a speech defect, being cross-eyed, labeled neurotic and hyperactive, beaten by adults, enduring short, sleepless nights, the emotional stripping of my sanity, sexual abuse, being forced to beat my twin brother, being physically restrained to eat food that I detested, spending endless hours locked away in foot lockers, receiving ruler beatings on my genitals from institutional supervisors, being forced to urinate and defecate, and subjected to constant verbal abuse by peers and instructors. These are true incidents in an unthinkable nightmare.

I was labeled a slow learner and was promptly placed in special education classes. I would spend the next eight years lost in a heap of bureaucratic red tape as well as teacher ignorance. My hunger for success and acceptance inspired me to overcome the physical and mental abuse that I would suffer over the years that lay ahead.

The summer of 1964 came and saw Jimmy and myself being placed in foster homes. Jimmy went to Three Rivers, while I went to Jackson, Michigan. After trial weekend situations with these families, we were preparing to leave many friends, but also to welcome new ones.

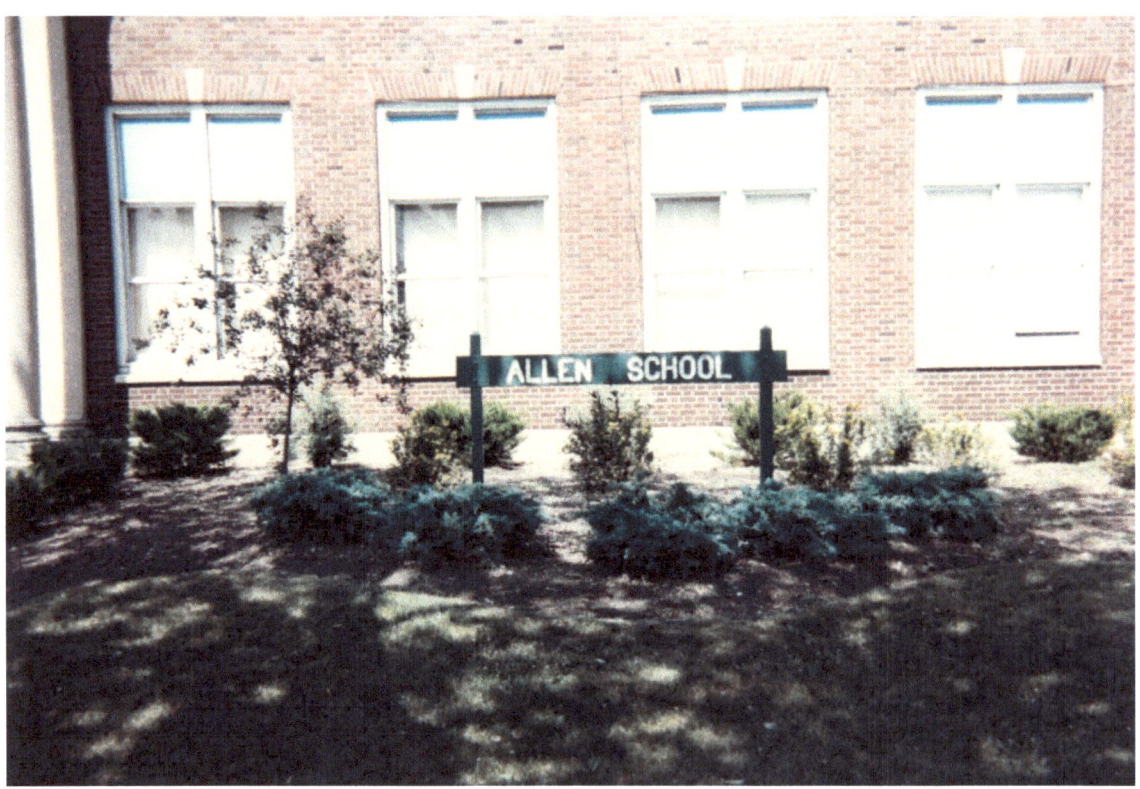

Above and Below: Allen Elementary School, now closed, was the first school I attended after being released from the Institution.

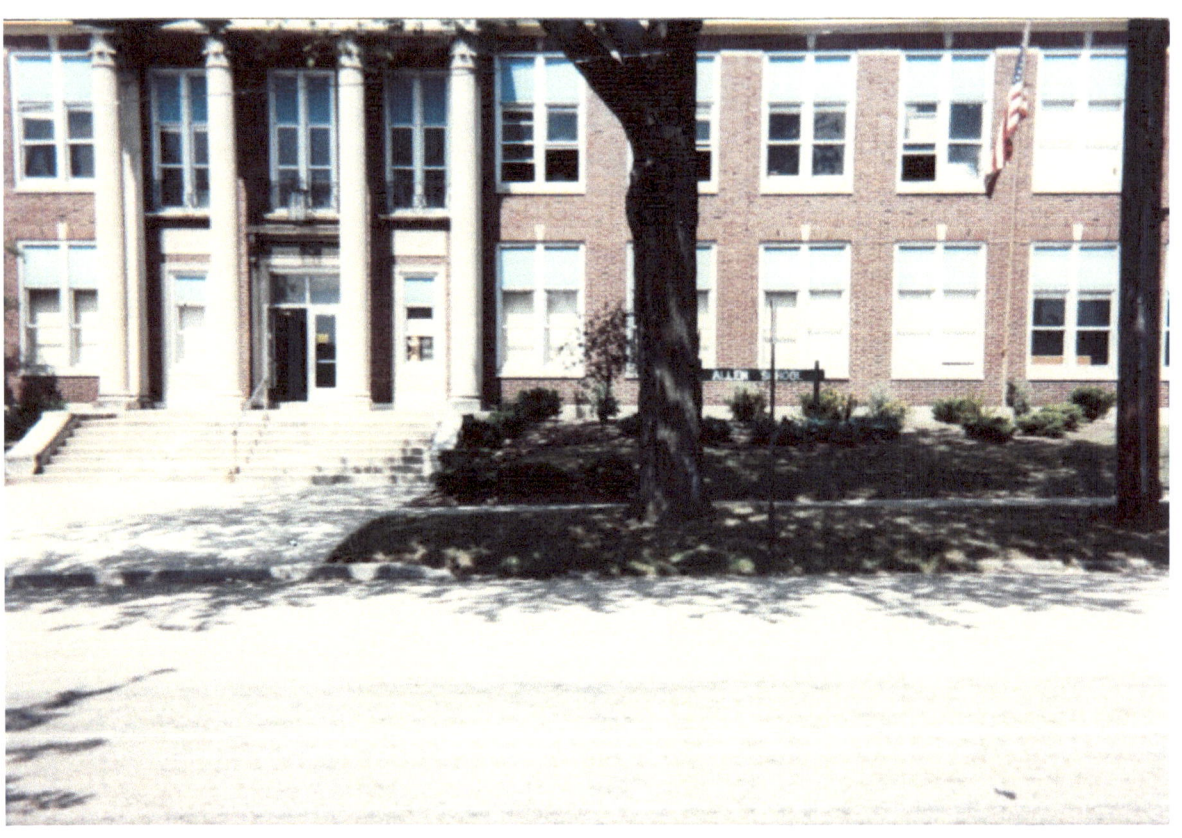

My New Home

The one hour drive that it took to get to Jackson from Coldwater seemed endless. It just didn't seem possible. After almost twelve years of being in boarding homes and institutions, I was going to a place that would be all my own.

My family seemed just as happy to see me as I was to see them. Leroy and Minnie Hinton were a hard working couple who had a grown son, David. He and his wife, Martha, had three children when I arrived which made me and uncle and first baby sitter. But after devouring everything in the refrigerator when babysitting, my new brother decided that it would be best to pay me rather than buy groceries after every night out.

The Hinton's welcomed me with a beautiful half German Shepard, half collie dog that I quickly named Buster. I had never owned a puppy before, so consequently, Buster and I became inseparable. Buster ate what I ate, and even slept in my bed, which drove my mother crazy. After formal greeting, I was off and running down the street to visit two old friends from Coldwater.

Charles and Andy had seen the dark station wagon pull up with me in it and were anxiously waiting for me to come visit them. Charles and Andy were responsible for my being placed here. Their foster parents, the Robinsons, talked with the Hinton's and then recommended me to be a foster care candidate. I was warmly welcomed to the neighborhood by the other kids and immediately felt that this was going to be a nice stay.

The summer of 1964 was long and hot. I quickly familiarized myself with my new surroundings by walking everywhere. Buster didn't seem to mind the walks either. My new family drove across town so that my Mom's sister could meet me. I was really impressed with my new cousin Larry. I think he must have been a prize fighter from those quick lefts and rights that he kept landing on my head! My new aunt, Victoria Austin, shouted to Larry, "Leave that boy alone, he's mentally retarded and doesn't know better." My cousin didn't care if I was dumb or not. All he knew was that if I opened my mouth again, there would be more of the same. I learned that life outside of Coldwater was not going to be as free as I once thought it would be.

The Allen Elementary School was across town from the local neighborhood school that I expected to attend. The new kids in class were similar to those in the class I attended at Coldwater, but I was soon to find out how cruel kids could be.

I was at least half a foot taller than most of the kids in school and became the target of "how is the weather up there?" and "Hello, Jolly Green Giant" jokes. Because of the condition of my eyes, I was called Clarence the Cross-Eyed Lion and Stagger Lips because of my speech problem.

Still school was going just fine. Again, as in Fort Custer, I had the attention of a teacher who took a great interest in me. However I was beginning to question the kind of attention given me and the other students. The touching and other advances made me uncomfortable. This went on for over a year in his home as well as at school. I felt unclean and was ashamed to tell anyone of this hidden secret that I would carry deep inside me for the next fifteen years. This was the second episode of my being sexually abused in twelve years, a tremendous burden of guilt for any twelve years old to carry around.

Dave Johnson, a tall man who visited our school during spring, invited me to try out for the basketball team after I was enrolled at the old East Junior High School in the fall. I was elated. This would be the first real athletic team that I had ever played on. East Junior High, when it was first built, was the largest school of its kind in the State of Michigan. The gymnasium where our basketball games were played was full to capacity. The noise and excitement were drowning out any instruction our coach hollered to us. I believed every one of our 800 plus student body was in attendance, especially when I scored my first basket! The joy of that first basket was too much for me, as it was for my teammates, because my two points went into the net of the other team! My first year on the team was otherwise uneventful, but the following years would see me lead the team to 19 straight wins and two championships.

My ninth grade year saw me captain of the football, basketball and track teams. It was in football that my most embarrassing moment occurred. My jock strap had just ripped apart, and I took a very large safety pin and pinned it together. I was leading our team in calisthenics when the pin came apart and stuck into my genitals! When Coach Young found out what I had done, that was the only time that I felt it was appropriate being call a moron.

I finally graduated from East Junior High School and looked forward to becoming a high school student. I also started a subscription to the Reader's Digest Book of the Month Club because my reading was on a fifth grade level, and I really wanted to improve in this area. I was receiving speech instruction and was recovering from my second eye operation. It was difficult adjusting to wearing eye glasses but it also felt great not to be the subject of jokes anymore. Bring on the Jackson High Vikings!

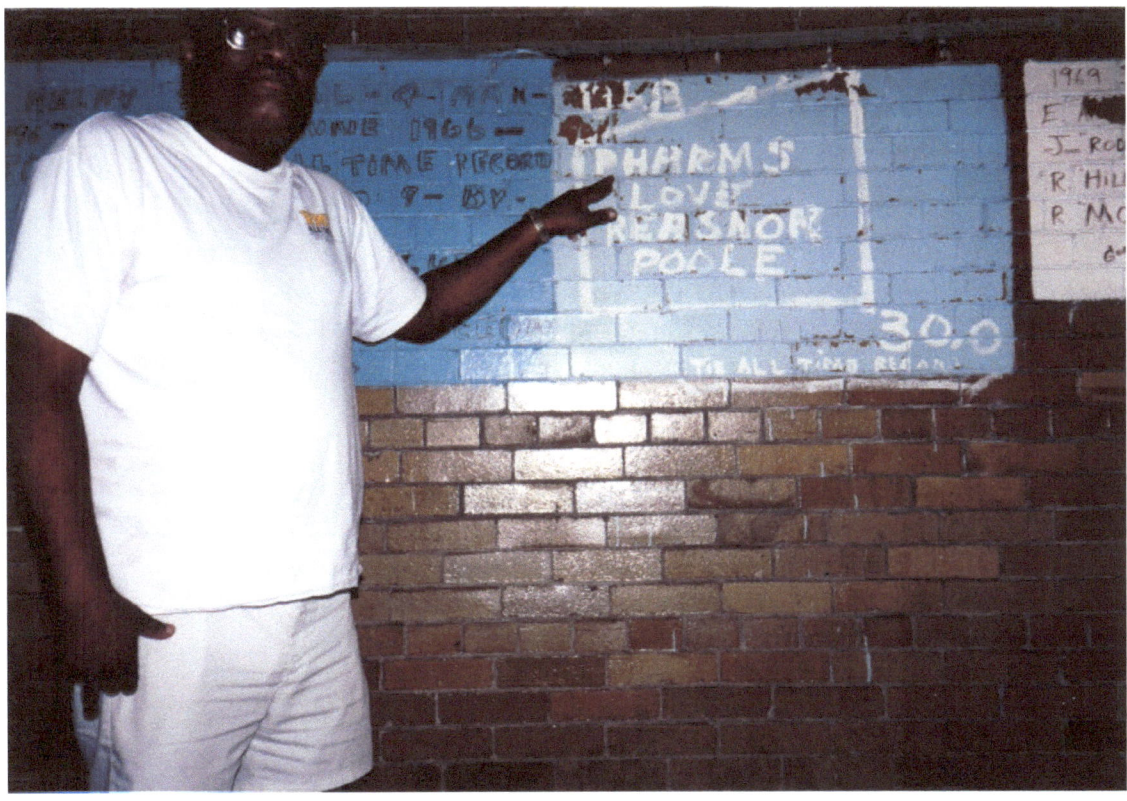

Above and Below: The wall of fame where I set many track records. This track was two levels above the basketball court!

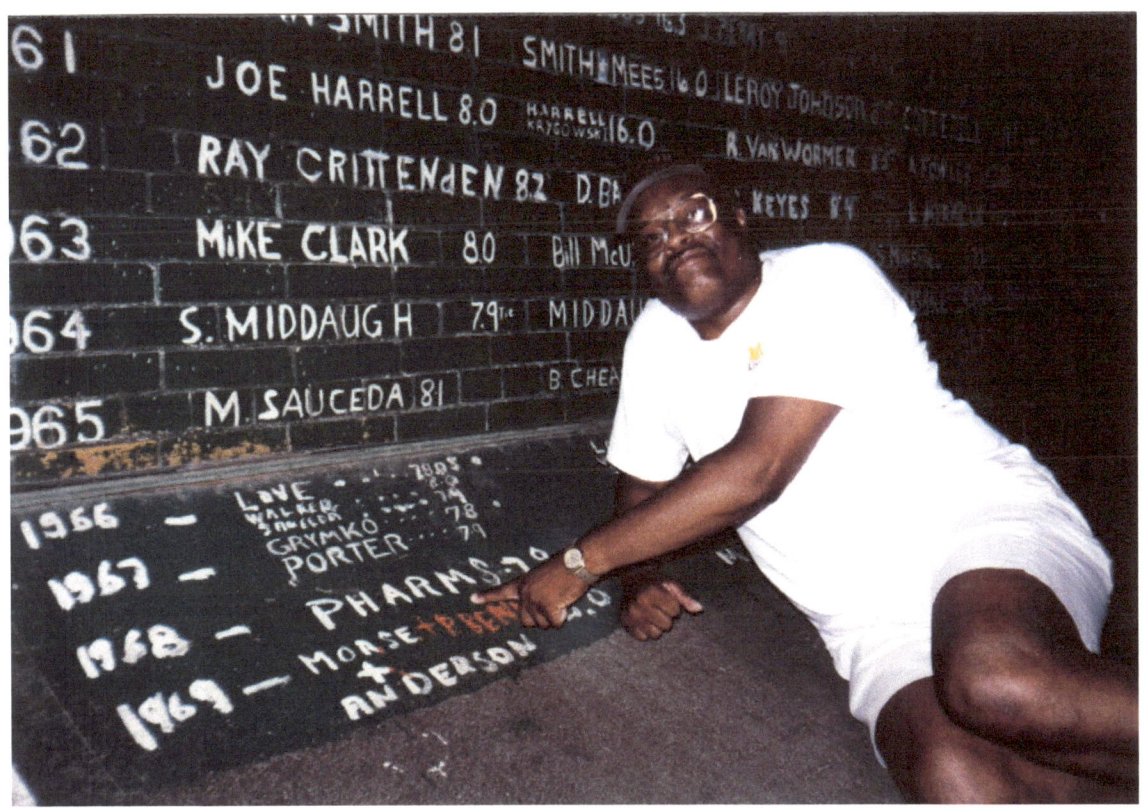

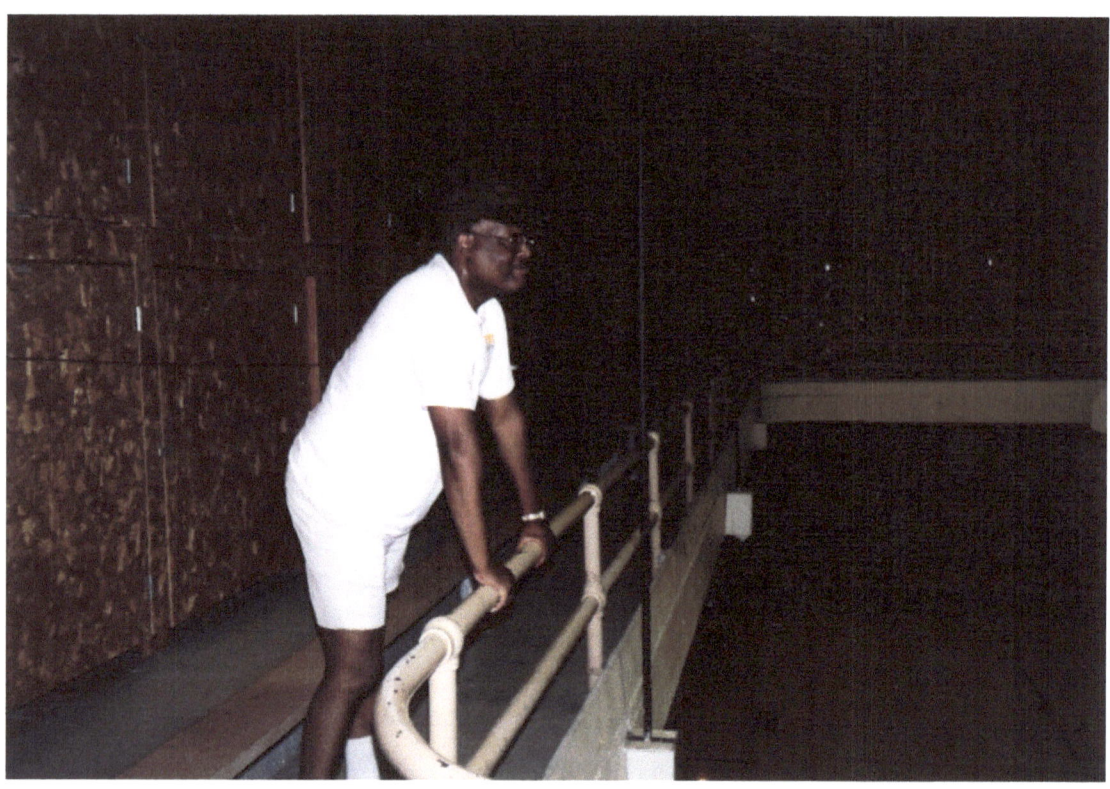

Above and Below: I'm looking down from the track, below are bleachers and below that the basketball court! Whew!

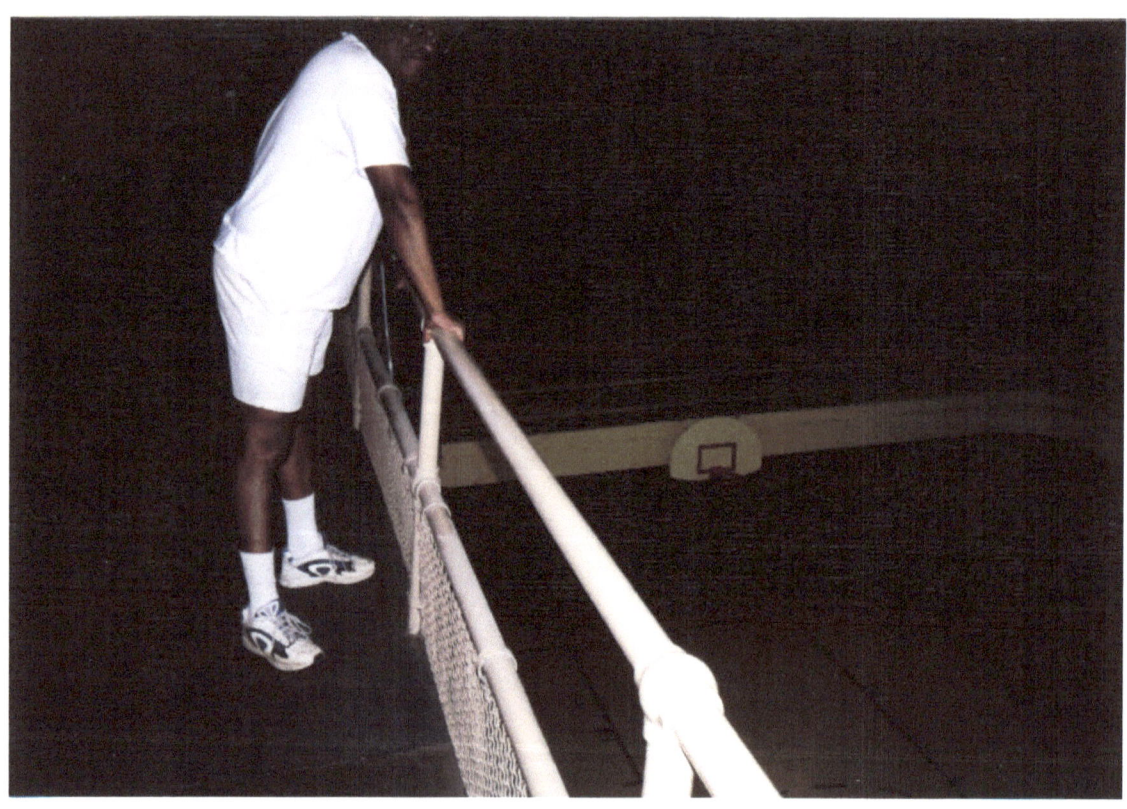

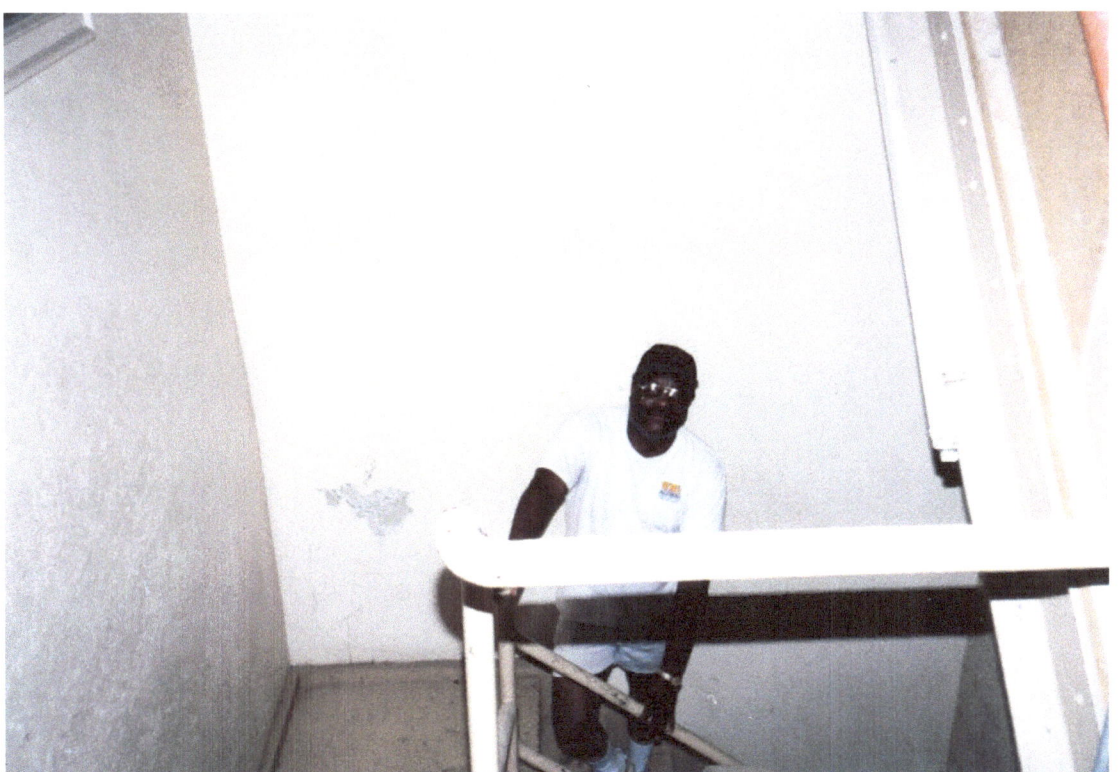

Heading down to the locker rooms from the basketball court.

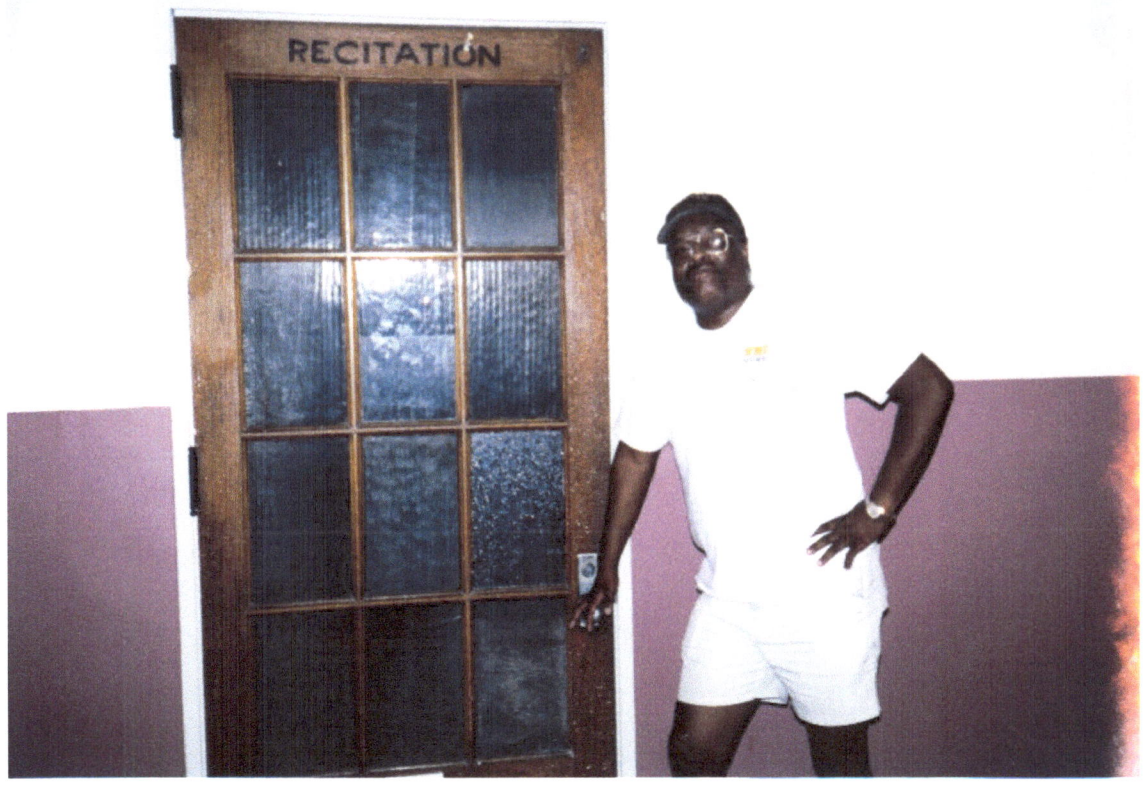

My old home room at the Junior High School

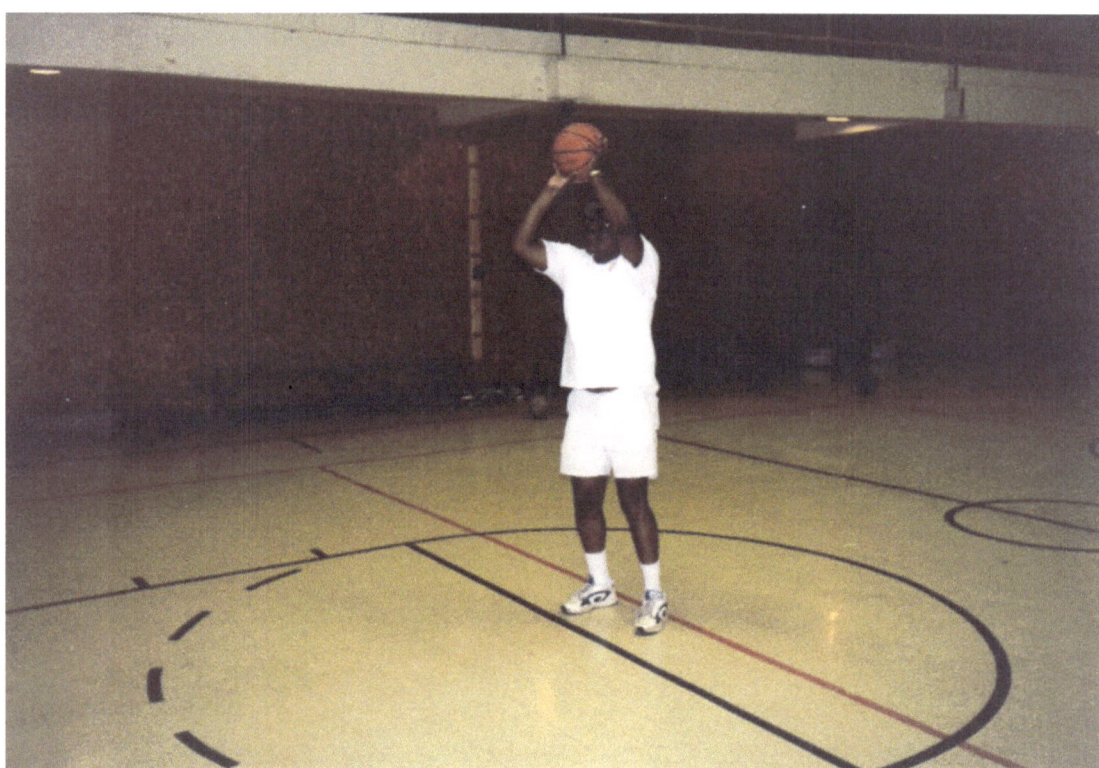

I'm taking a shot on the very same floor where our Junior High School team remained undefeated for two years running. We even beat the teachers.

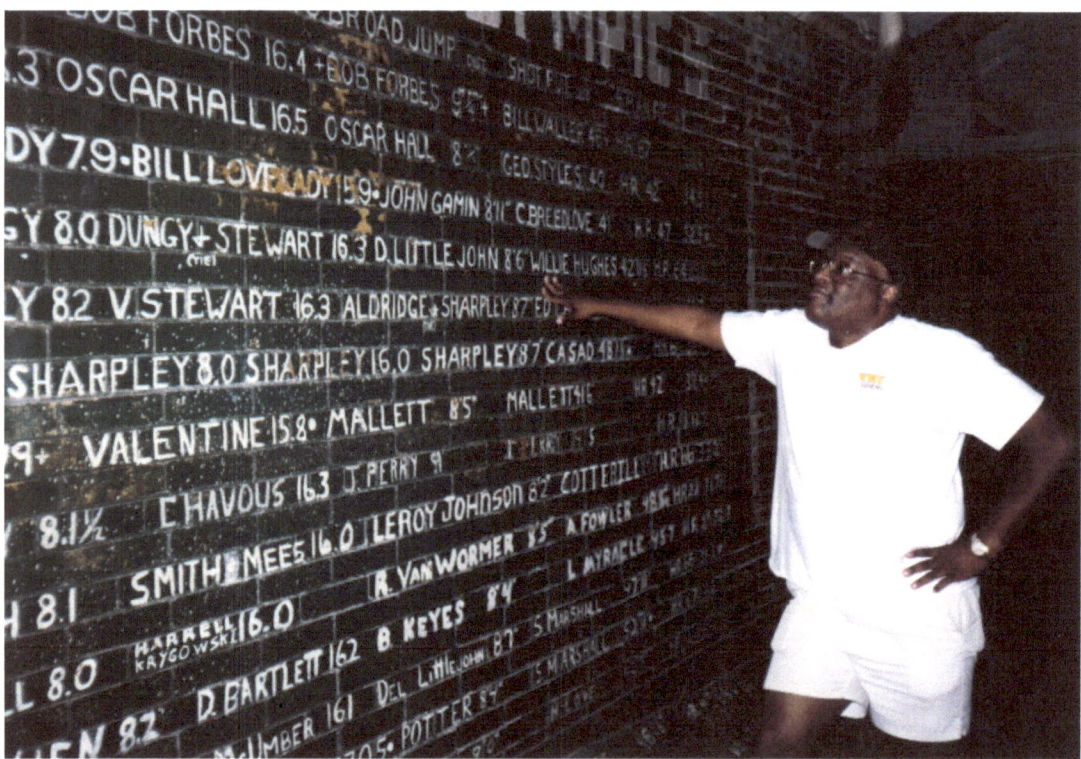

The wall of fame where I set many track records. This track was two levels above the basketball court!

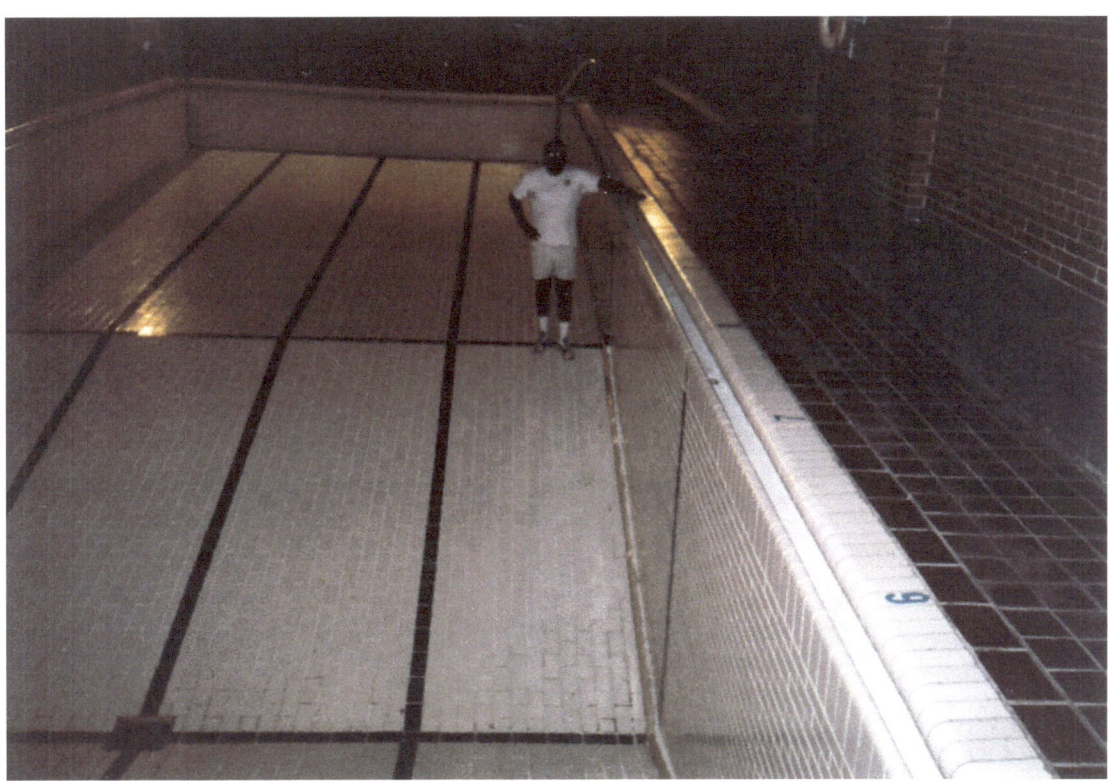

Above and Below: I'm standing in the middle of the Jr. High School's pool where I once swam four lengths underwaters.

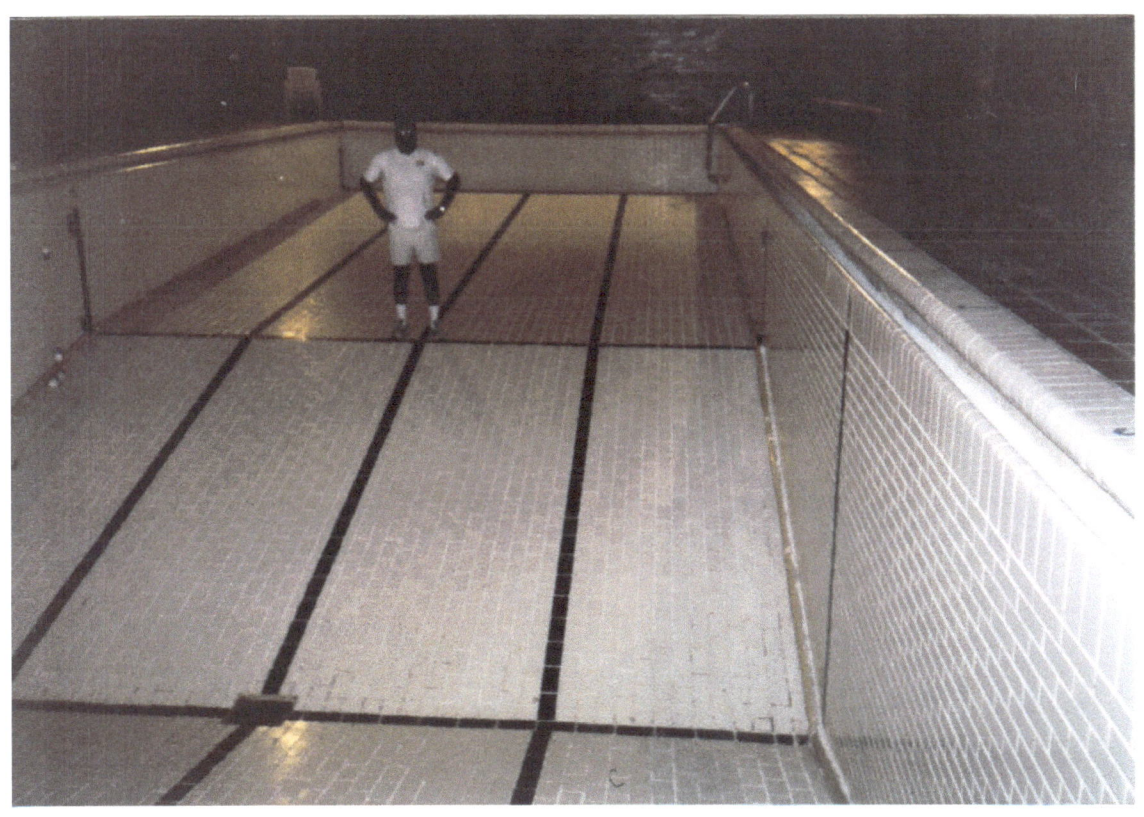

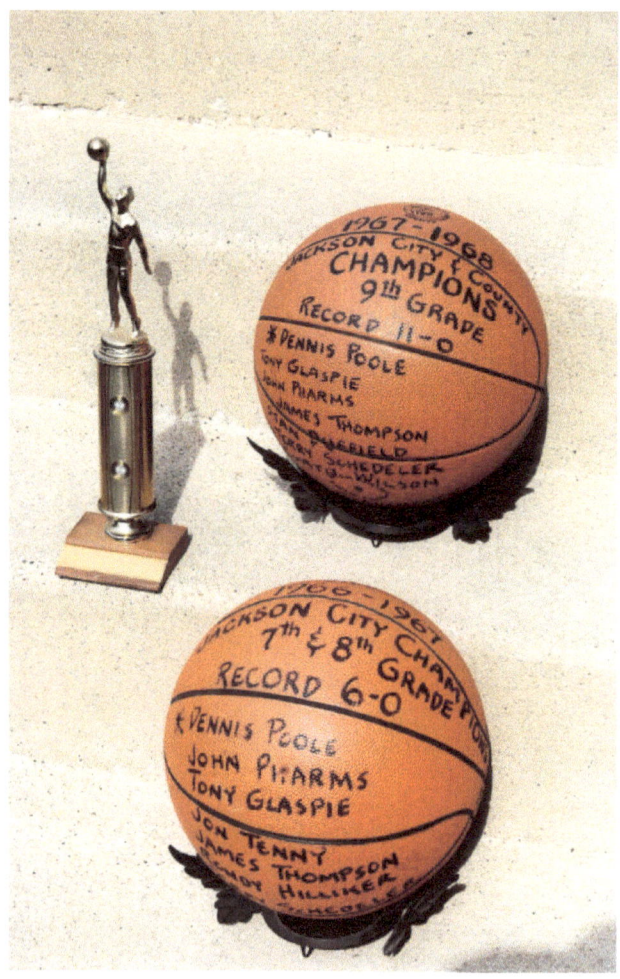

Below: I'm Standing the gym of the institution that is now a Michigan Prison

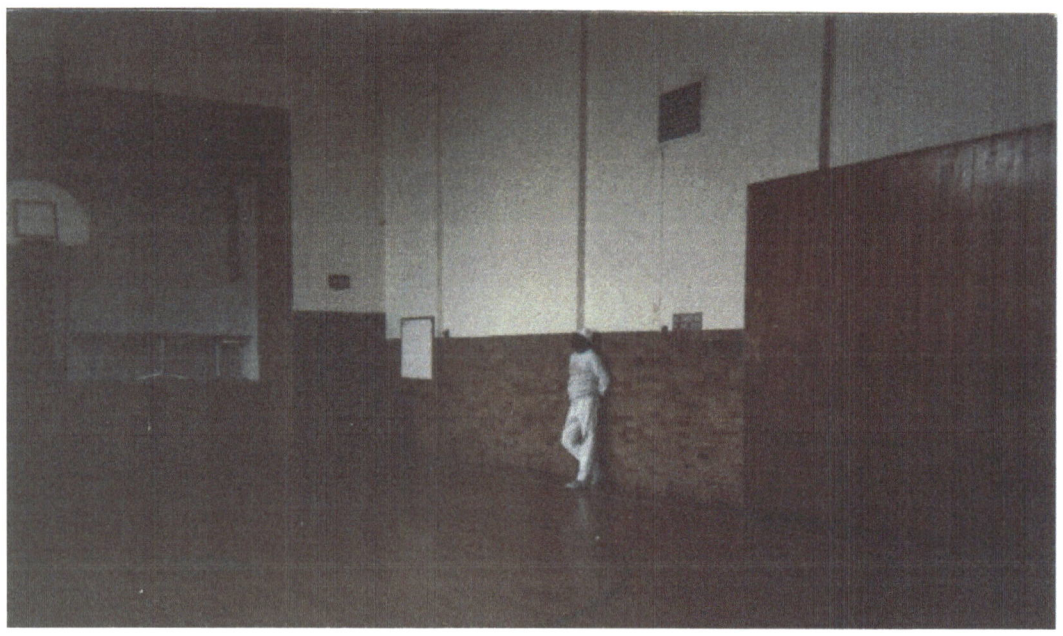

School and Coping With My Abusive Parents

Now my new parents were definitely not the same sweet, loving family that they were when we first met. Their attitude change was something that I had to adjust to. If my chores were not completed to their satisfaction, they would threaten me by dialing the number to Coldwater.

Once, after I criticized a eacher for lying to me, he informed my mom. My mom gave me a beating with a razor strap and kept hitting me until I started to cry. The last time I had cried was the first beating in Coldwater. The marks from that day are still reminders to me of the many beatings I endured.

My parents fought with each other often. It always seemed to be over drinking or Dad gambling away his check. Shouting matches were very common. Physical attacks and flying objects were a weekly ritual. But whenever my social worker arrived for a home visit, the best foot forward was the order of the day. Even with the financial support from Coldwater and the constant borrowing of my allowance by my Dad, my parents seemed to be constantly broke.

I remember one chilling day when my Dad came home, loaded his .35 caliber revolver and went back to the South Side Club to get back the money he lost while gambling. That scene frightened me. Seeing your Dad come home with cuts on his head and leaving with a gun in his hand would scare most children. Mom had to always put off buying the groceries until Dad had money. Not eating didn't bother me so much, but when the Probate Court of Grand Rapids finally took custody of me, they found that I had been undernourished.

School became a support system for me. My future goal of attending college depended upon my graduating from high school. I kept saying to myself, how was this going to come about with me still attending special education classes and having a reading deficiency? After years of Dick and Jane type materials, I made the bold but crucial decision to enroll in regular high school classes. This decision would not hold well with my teachers, social worker, or family. My social worker felt that I had overestimated my athletic and intellectual abilities. My grade counselor and my social worker believed that I was receiving as much instruction as students taking regular courses, and they also believed that I would be intimidated by more academic competition, but this was one competition that I was determined I would work hard to win.

The Jackson High School football team, once a state power, had fallen on hard times. My sophomore year was also marred with racial unrest. Our school experienced two large riots during the years. To make things even worse, during our homecoming game our athletic director died on the field. We finished that year with a record of 0-9.

Going into my junior year, I had already established myself on the athletic field. During my junior year we were determined to win more than our share of games. We started off well as we won our opening game, but we proceeded to lose our next eight games and finished with a record of 1-8 that year.

The 1970 Viking season opened with great expectations. We were alive with emotions not seen on our campus in years. We defeated Tony Dungy's Parkside Eagles for the first time in eight years in front of over 8,000 screaming fans. Tony would go on to play and coach for the Pittsburg Steelers while his mother would be the first instructor at our school who totally believed in me. Our team finished with a record of 7-2 for the year, which would represent the school's best year since 1944. We also won the city championship.

Basketball season was different. After arriving from East Junior High School having enjoyed two years of success, I was ready for the high life. My sophomore year was fair, but I was let go from the team during my junior year. I would later be asked to try out for the basketball team at Western Michigan University by former Ohio State Basketball Coach Edlon Miller. After college, I would play on teams for five years in Spain and Denmark.

Track was my best sport. I ran on the Varsity team for three years. I co-captained the team in my senior year, when I also qualified for the state meet in the 440 yard dash.

With my athletic career over, I now faced the biggest challenge of my life.

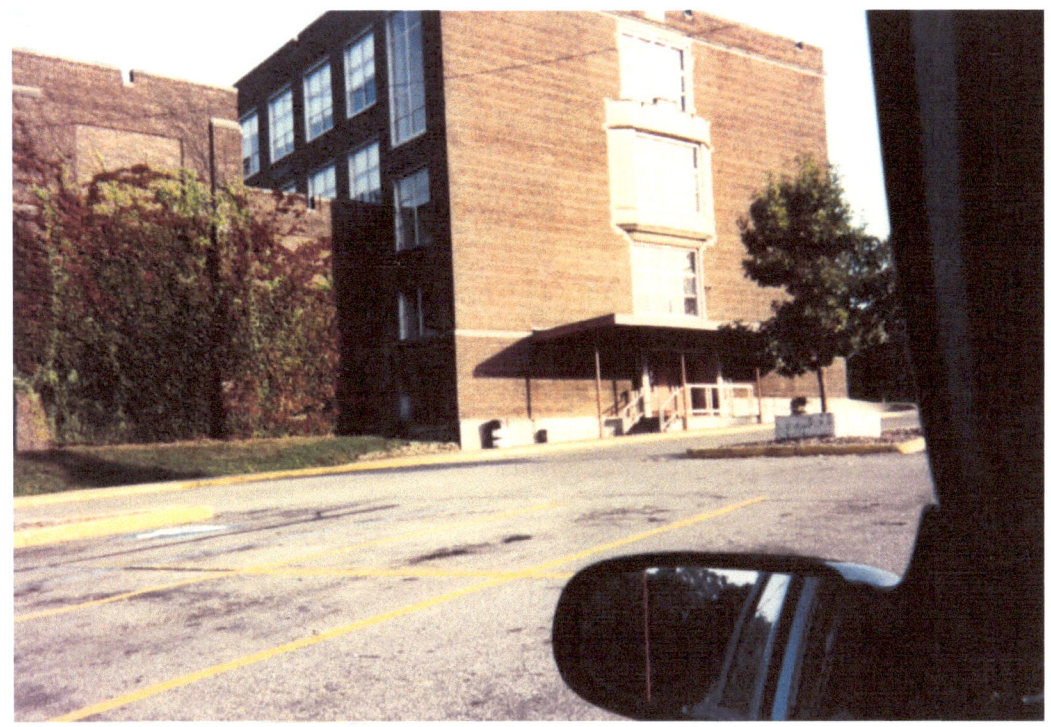

Above and Below: Jackson High School. Home of the Vikings!

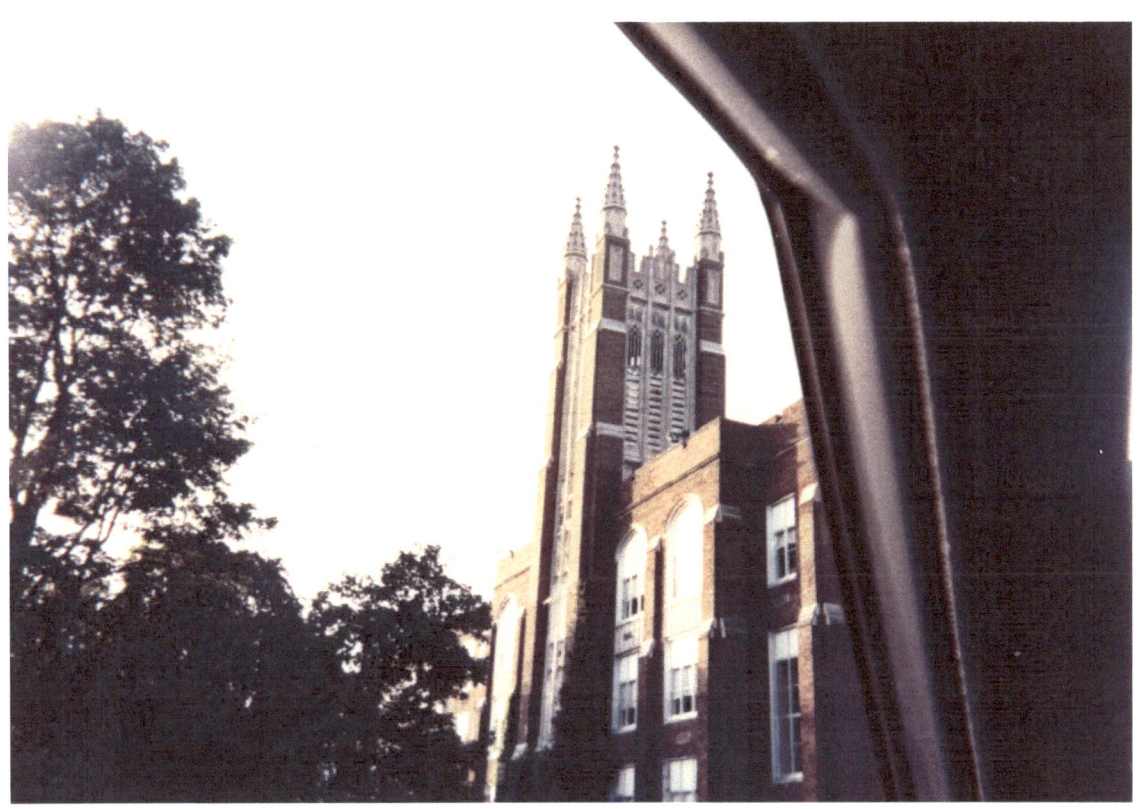

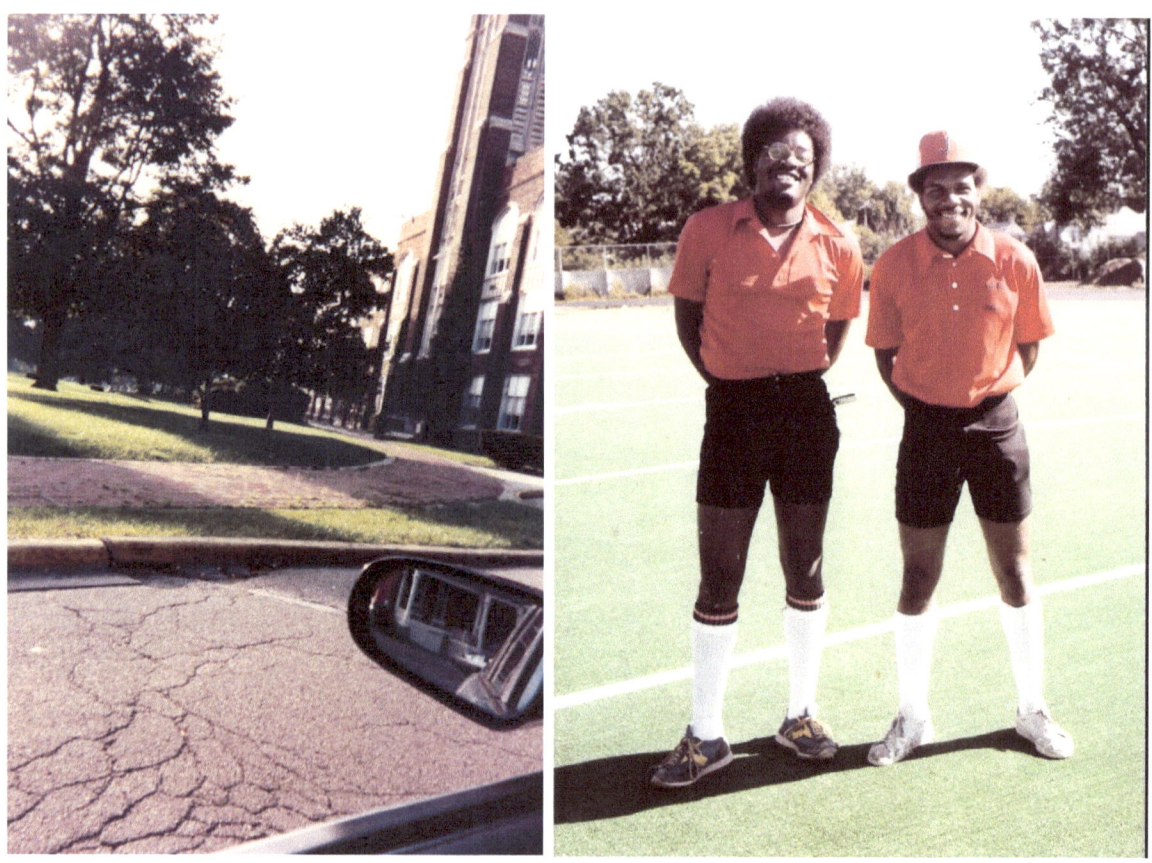

Top Left: Jackson High School. Home of the Vikings! *Top Right*: I'm standing with my close friend Rickey Oliver. I was the head freshman football coach and Rickey was the quarterback coach *Below:* This is me running to the finish line for Jackson High School.

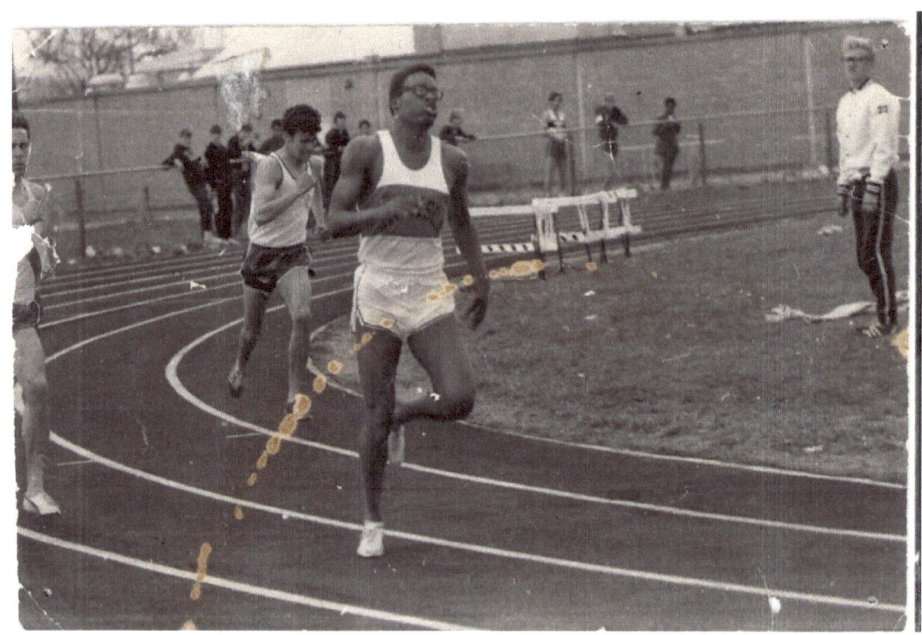

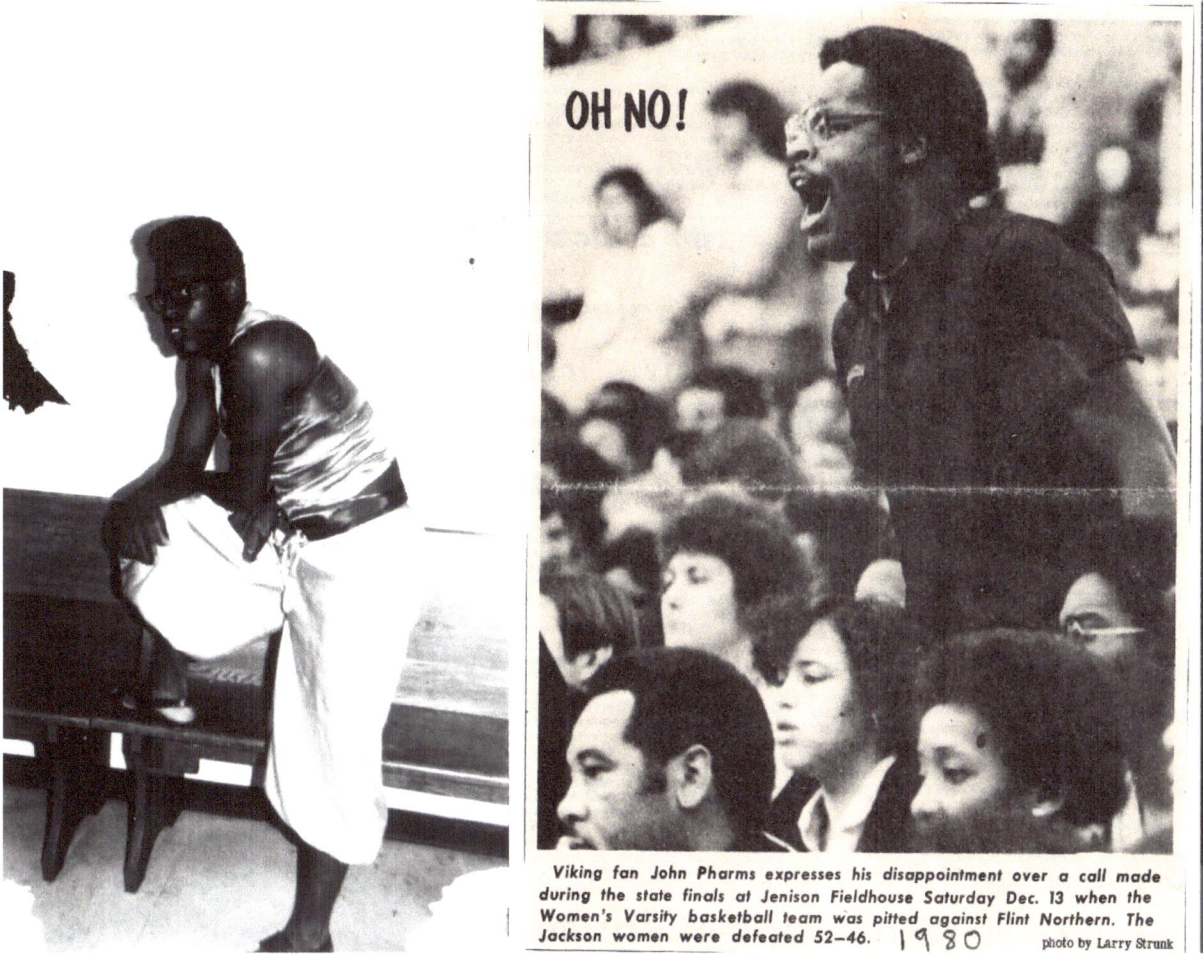

OH NO!

Viking fan John Pharms expresses his disappointment over a call made during the state finals at Jenison Fieldhouse Saturday Dec. 13 when the Women's Varsity basketball team was pitted against Flint Northern. The Jackson women were defeated 52—46. 1980   photo by Larry Strunk

Top Left: This is me preparing for the small school production of the King and I with me as the King! *Top Right*: Vikings fan John Pharms expresses his disappointment over a call made during the sate finals at Jenison Fieldhouse Saturday Dec. 13 when the Women's Varsity basketball team was pitted against Flint Northern. The Jackson women were defeated 52-46.

The Untold Yet Remarkable Story of a Very Determined Little Boy Named Johnnie

While still diagnosed as mental retarded, I wrote this poem in the tenth grade:

Let's Get It All Together

Get together America
Or die by the cross
Get together America
We have not yet lost.

Love that man because he's your friend
Love that man and by the
Color of his skin.

Put it all together.
Or pay the price,
Unite my fellow brother
Don't gamble with your life.

Air pollution, garbage, and
Polluted waters,
America the beautiful?
I don't think so.

We have to get together
And learn to help one another
We have to reach out
And help our land.

Old folks and old ways
Sorry madam and sir
But not in this modern day
It's young people and new ways.

God created the heaven and the earth
God created love and faith
But who created hate and sin?
Satan and his evil men.
People who criticize those who fight
Finding dead bodies still
In the night.
Blacks and whites are off to war
Man is on his way to a third
World War.
Build up the slums and
Help the poor.
Let's get it all together and

End all wars.
Pretty soon now it could mean war.

Americanis the world power;
America has the government power
America shall soon be dead
Unless we learn to hold up our heads.
Foreign countries love our beauty
Foreign people come to stay
Beauty could shine from day to day
If only man could learn to keep it
That way.

The black man deprived of his dignity
A whole century of white man's lies
They say, say it loud. I'm black and
I'm proud.
Man has fooled all people
He's like a clown with make-up on his face,
He fools those who can only hope and
Pray or visualize a reality of love.
And freedom for men, black and white
Pretty soon now he must unmask his face,
And say proudly, "I am an American"

Don't fear communism!
Fight it!
Don't fear drugs and dope!
Fight it!
Don't fear man and his evil weapons!
Fight It!
Fight him with something he does not know,
Fight him with Christianity,
Fight him with what you know
Not what you hear or see.
If we can get it all together,
Then we shall have power
A power of "One nation, under God
Indivisible with liberty and justice for all."
Because we are all human.

The Untold Yet Remarkable Story of a Very Determined Little Boy Named Johnnie

The Plot

My social worker had a long discussion with my parents indicating that it was time for them to bring me down to earth. They were told to make me realize that it takes a great deal of ability to be able to go to college, and it was very doubtful that I would be able to pass a college examination. They felt my aspirations for wanting to achieve as much as possible were good and they wanted me to think this, but they also believed I was aiming for an impossible goal. They felt that they should talk to me regarding what type of special education/vocational training course I should take during my last two years of high school. They discussed with me the nature of special education classes and they pointed out the fact that I was receiving much of the same material that regular high school students were receiving, but that this material was not presented to me as fast because I would not learn as much.

My grade counselor made an appointment with my placement coordinator about either a special education co-op program or a special education work experience program. My grade counselor became annoyed with me as I had signed up for regular classes on my own. I was determined to make it either face down or standing up.

By this time, Mrs. Dunny was giving me all of the confidence that I needed to take me to the next level of higher learning. I overcame all of these obstacles to accept the Martin Luther King Jr. Scholarship to attend Western Michigan University. Nelson Jackson and Roger Pullian, representative of the scholarship program, were as excited as I was, and they felt that I would do quite well at Western Michigan. Even now my social worker had become a believer in my determination to succeed.

The Discharge

"John has been under the jurisdiction of the court and/or institution for the mentally retarded since shortly after one year of age."

"John has been attending the Jackson Public Schools since his family care in 1964. He received his diploma from Jackson High School in1971."

"I am recommending that John Pharms be discharged from the jurisdiction of the Coldwater State Home and Training School."

I was happy to be leaving my foster care home. My foster parents were difficult to live with. Many nights, after a weekend of drinking, they would come home fighting. This was typical of them during the seven years I was living with them. No more fights and, for the first time in almost twenty years of living, no more restrictions! College was going to be fun. Just as I had imagined while watching the *Ozzie and Harriet* television show! Nothing could stop me now.

Yes, There Really Is A Kalamazoo

College was going to be different: no more curfews and no more restrictions. College life was going to be everything that I had dreamed of. I was aiming to make up for a lot of lost time.

I was not prepared for the arrival of so many students. Western Michigan University had an enrollment of over 21,000 students. The main campus which included the athletic dormitory was to be my first home away from home. French Hall was an athletes' dormitory that housed Fall, Winter and Spring athletes. I was preparing to try out for the football team when I met my roommate. Ben was huge: 6'5" tall and weighing over 250 pounds. He became my first best friend. We would do most things together and what made this union so unusual was that Ben was white.

Our campus was going through tremendous racial unrest. The year before I arrived at Western, a black student was shot by a white officer, and this touched off a bitter resentment between blacks and whites. We also had anti-Vietnam demonstrations on our campus just like every other campus across America. This was not supposed to be happening, I told myself. Where was the fun? I had enrolled in college to have fun.

Then came my first letter from Uncle Sam. I had no uncle name Sam. I had never hit the lottery either until that day. My luck was changing. The letter from Uncle Sam was a rude awakening to the reality of life. The Vietnam War had become a very unpopular war that America was no longer willing to accept. My lottery number was fifteen, which meant that in two years I would serve my country. My academics were suffering, and I had begun to doubt if I even belonged in college. Maybe, everybody was correct. Maybe, I just didn't belong there. But I kept pushing on.

Are You My Real Mom?

Chuck and Miriam Sargent, not to be confused with my foster family, were a very warm and caring couple. They were more than just friends to me. With children of their own, they always treated me as part of their immediate family beginning during my younger years. They treated me like a real son, and I treated them like my real parents. No one else has treated me more like a son than they did. Chuck and Miriam befriended me during the time when I needed a real family. For seven years, they were there. Yet, I still had this feeling that I had to know the truth. I still had to know my parents.

The telephone operator gave me the telephone number of a Frank Pharms who was my real uncle. Frank and his wife drove over from Grand Rapids to meet me and take me to visit my Mom. It took the weekend before I finally decided to go to meet my Mom. I crossed the street where my uncle had parked and walked up the twelve steps to my Mom's house. This small, dark, blood-eyed woman didn't know who I was. She opened the door, and we stood staring at each other. After twenty years of hatred, the wait was over. So was the visit. I couldn't wait to get back to campus. I decided then that meeting my Dad, who lived in Houston, could wait.

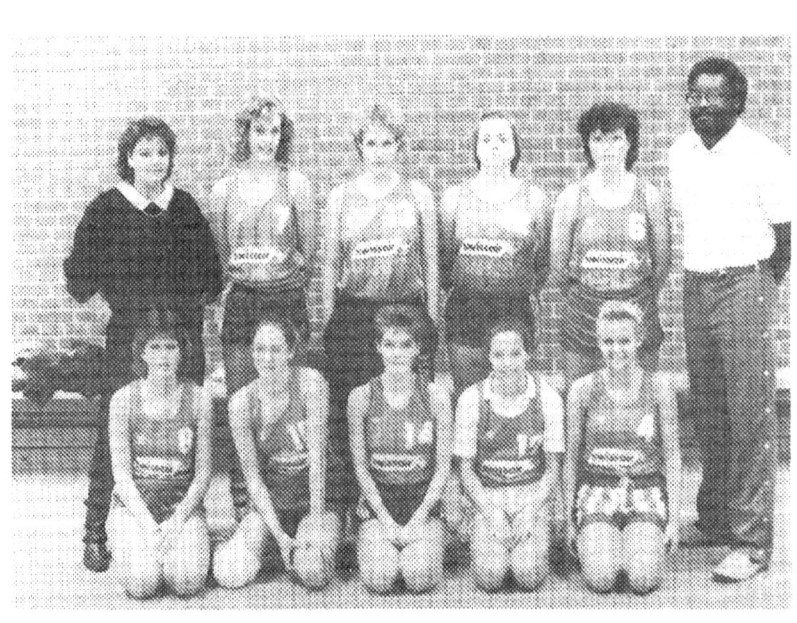

Above and Below: This is me while I was a teacher and head basketball in Holstobro, Demark 1985-87.

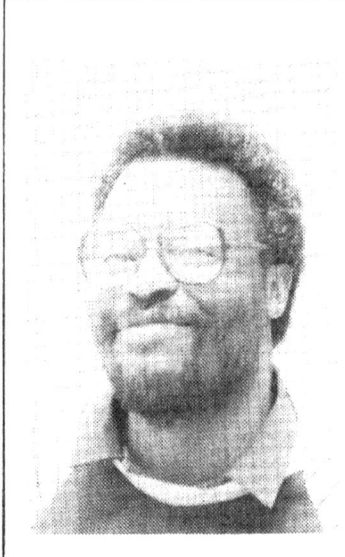

Coach : John Pharms.

Uddannet på Western Michigan University i 1977 og har siden da beskæftiget sig med mange former for sport og undervisning i bl.a. løb, amerikansk fodbold, atletik, fysisk træning og basketball. Før John kom til Danmark i 1985, var han idrætslærer på den amerikanske skole på Mallorca. I Harlev var John sidste år træner for drenge- og pigeholdet, mens han i år tager sig af de bedste damer.

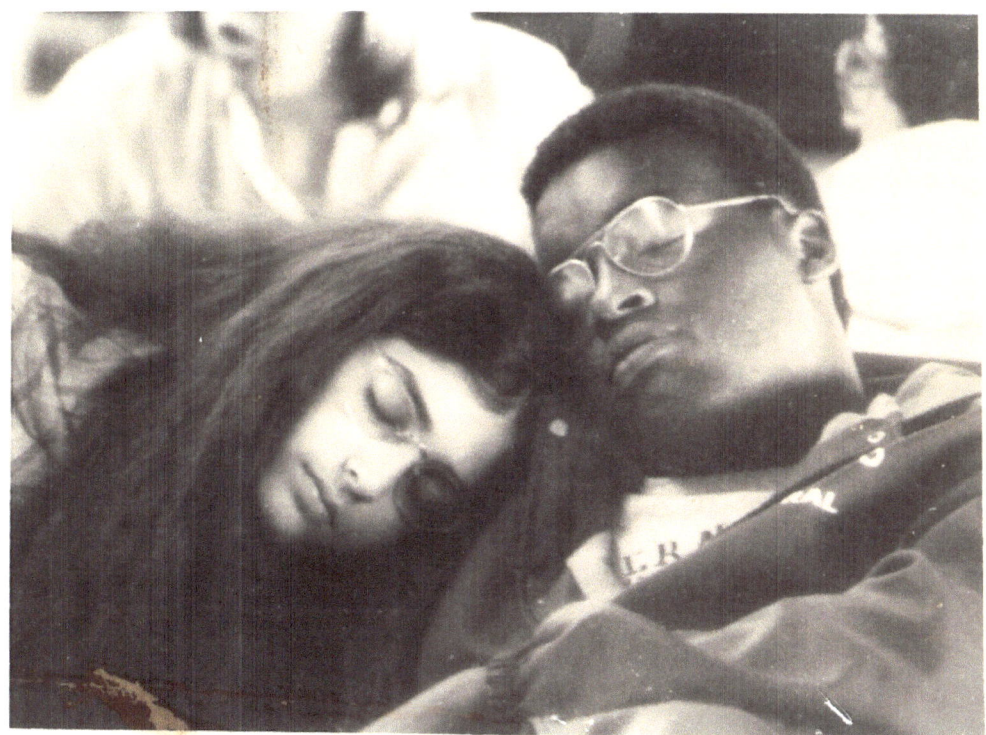

This is me with my friend Aimee as we take a short nap waiting for our flight to Denmark as exchange students.

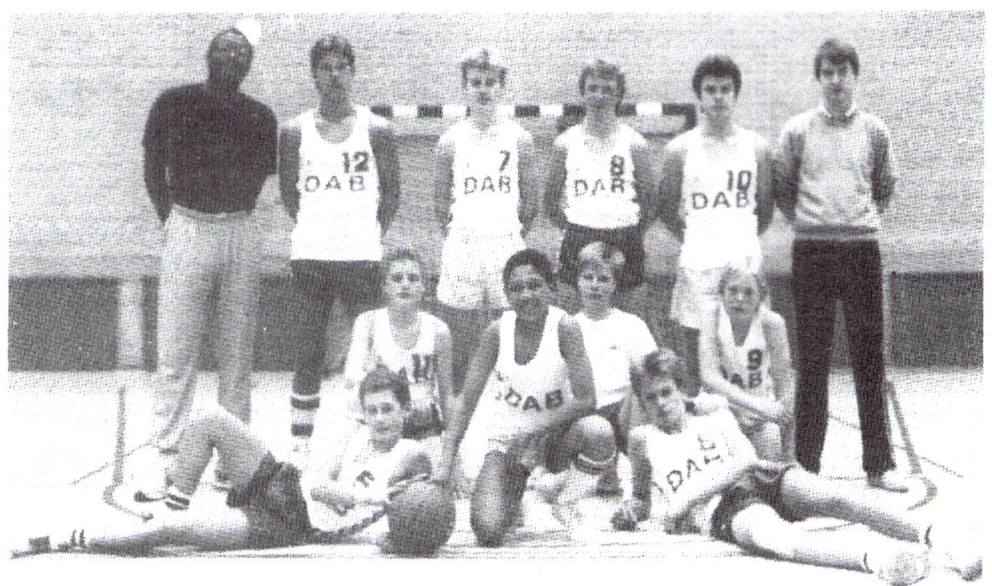

Drengene blev nr. 2 ved DM. Her ses en del af spiller-truppen samt John L. Pharms og Ove.

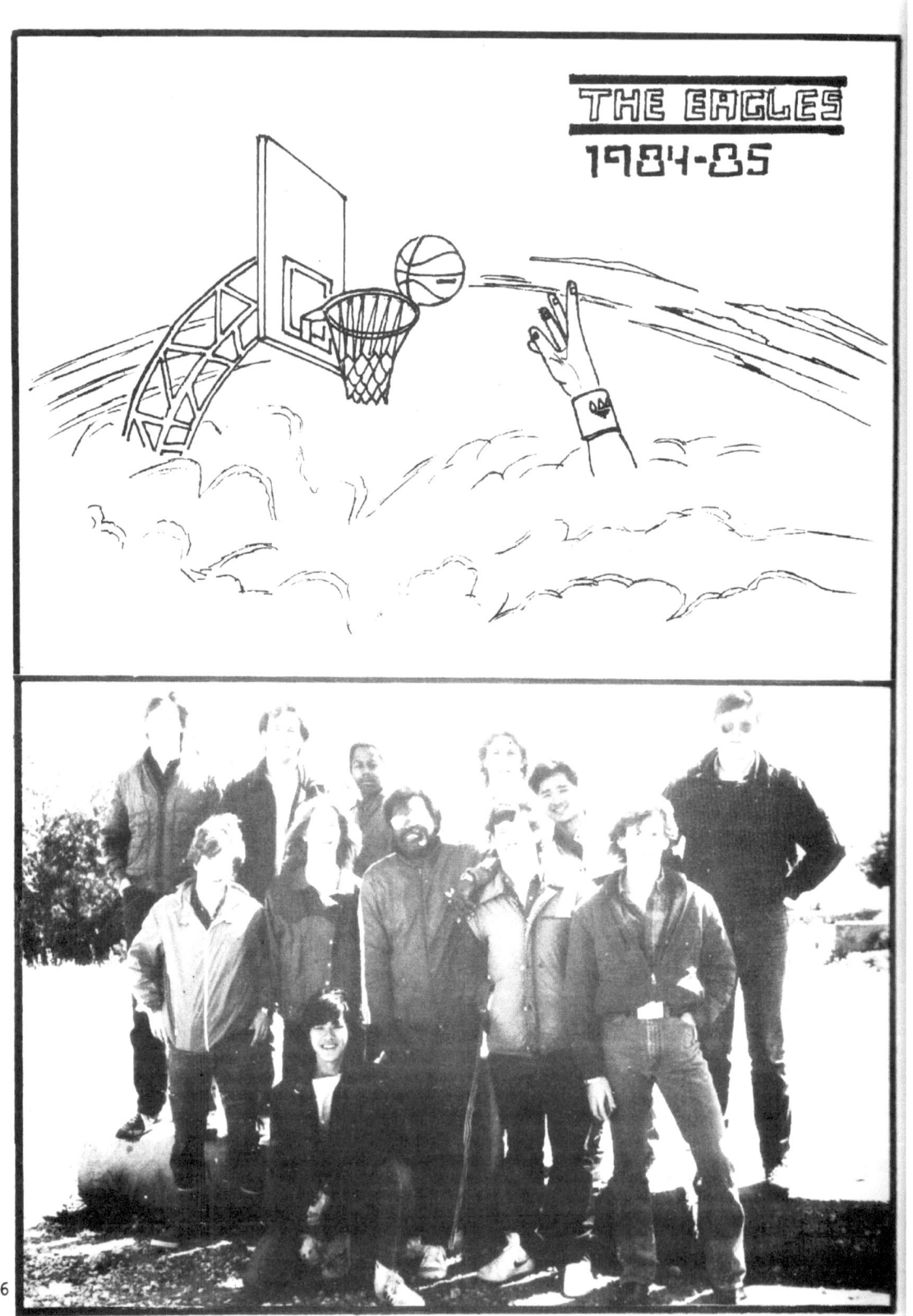

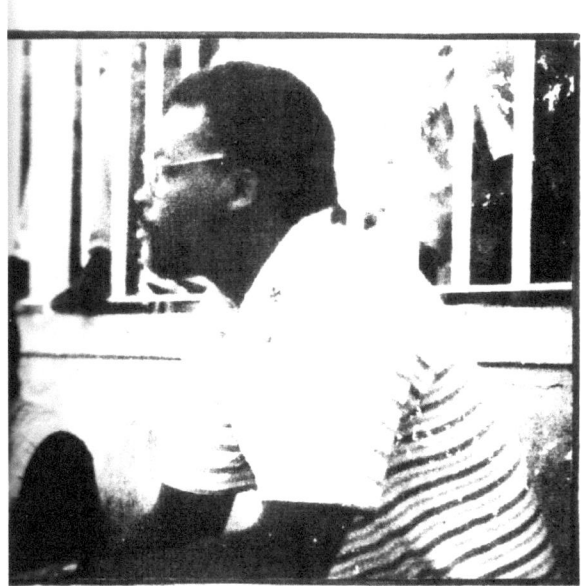

ASM	OPPONENTS	OPPONENTS
	Barcelona Tournament	
66	Barcelona-Abad-Oliba	39
39	ASM Barcelona	45
	League Season	
74	C.I.D.E.	66
55	LaSalle	48
96	Alcudia	49
56	San Jose	96
75	Perlas	39
68	C.I.D.E.	72
80	ASM Faculty	60
101	LaSalle	72
62	San Jose	95
57	LLuchmayor	58
66	Alcudia	33
70	LLuchmayor	76
2	La Puebla (Forfeit)	0
2	Alcudia (Forfeit)	0
89	Perlas	61
79	Ramon LLull	85
62	Juan Capo	65
72	Perlas	58
66	La Puebla	46
100	Alcudia	49
2	Ramon LLull (Foefeit)	0
2	Perlas (Foefeit)	0
2	Juan Capo (forfeit)	0
	Madrid Tournament	
67	ASM Barcelona	37
48	A.I.S. Lisbon (Portugal)	34
71	ASM Madrid	105

19 Wins   9 Losses

SEASON SUMMARY 1984-85

The curtain has fallen on the 1984-85 American School of Mallorca basketball season and it is time for us to reflect some of the great moments in Eagle history.

The season got off to a rather disappointing start as the Eagles lost to ASM-Barcelona in their tournament on the mainland by a score of 45-39. The Eagles won their earlier match against Barcelona-Abad-Oliba by a score of 66-39.

The Eagles returned home to begin league action in hopes of improving upon last year's league mark of 10 wins and 6 loses and their overall record of 16-7 which was capped off by their 56-54 victory over ASM Madrid that was played in Madrid, Spain.

Marty Bennett and Howard Morgan were back to lead a revamp offense led by new guard James Thomas. The Eagles roared by their first three opponents setting up a conference showdown with San Jose. The Eagles lost to San Jose who went on to represent Mallorca to decide the overall champion in Spain. The Eagles, however, did surpass last year's school record. (League) of 10 and finished with 15 and an overall record of 19-9 for the year.

The Eagles traveled to Madrid, Spain to defend the Liberal Cup won over ASM Madrid last year by a score of 55-51. The Eagles made it to the championship round, but lost to ASM Madrid 105-71.

Graduating from this year's team are Matt Reager, Cees Teljer, Matt Morgan, Chris Cannon and school record holders Marty Bennett (1,808 career points) and Howard Morgan (career record holder for rebounds in a season with 411). Randy Russell, who finished the season as the most improved player, is transferring to another school for his senior year.

The Eagles finished the year with a school record 19 wins. Coach Pharms, once again, has made the Eagles a formidable opponent in the Spanish Basketball League. Coach Pharms has a two year career record here at ASM of 35 wins and 16 loses.

And to the fighting ASM Eagles, we say thank you and much success

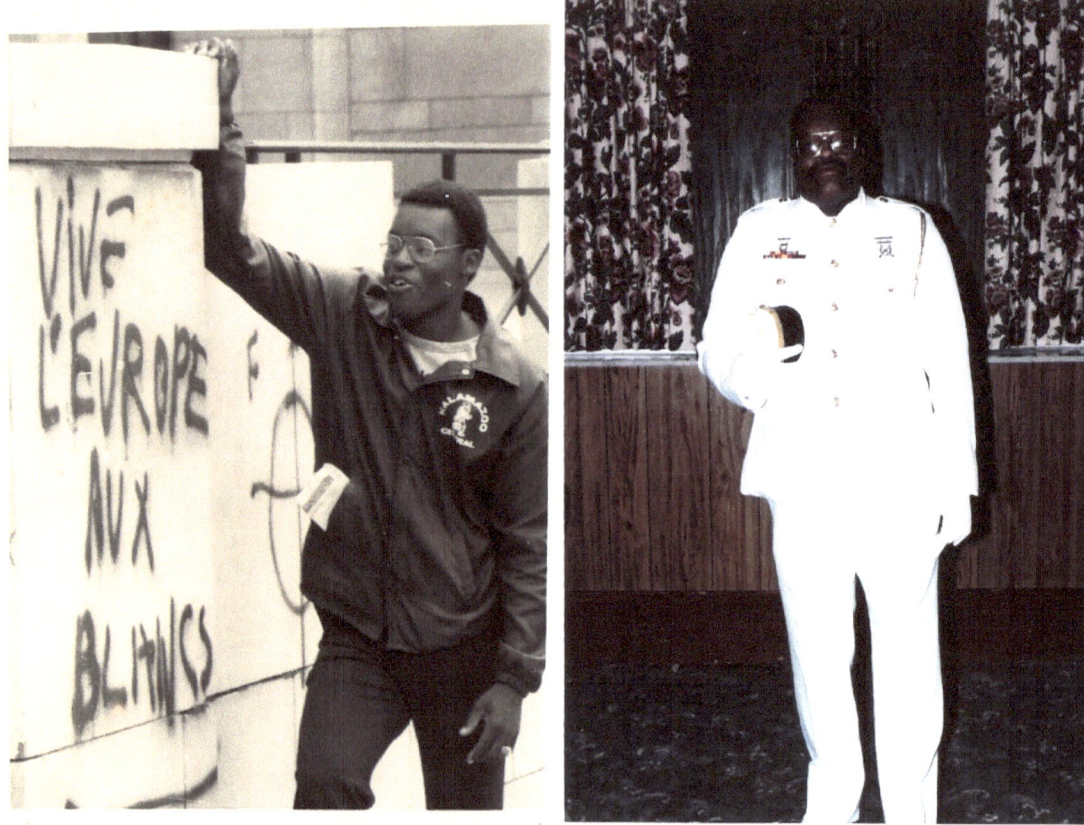

Top Left: I took French in college at Western Michigan University and if you can read this you know what it says. *Top Right:* I'm at a dinner reception as Captain of the Titanic. I do NOT plan on going down with the ship! *Below:* This is me as a Teacher, Athletic Director, House Father and Coach on the Island of Mallorca, Spain 1983-85.

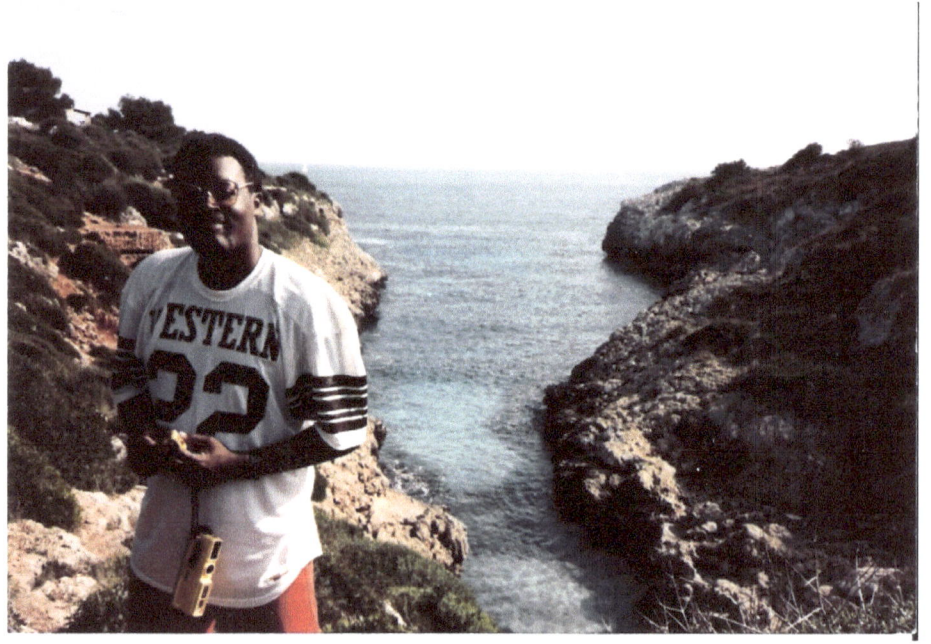

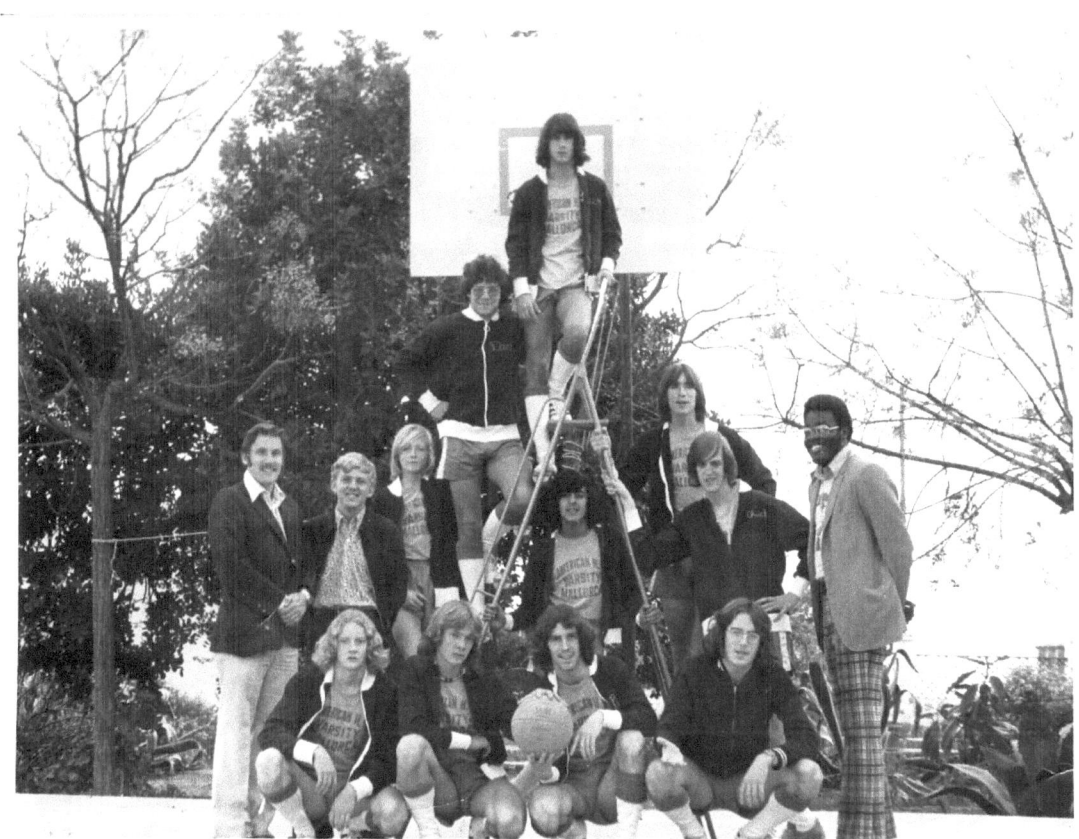

This is me (right side standing) with my high school basketball team on the Island of Palma De Mallorca, Spain 1974.

Epilogue

I graduated from Western Michigan, and with that degree came the realization that I had finally made it:I had achieved my goal. Twenty-five years have passed, and I've finally erased the memory of all those institutions and years of being treated as a mentally retarded person.

I went back to my old high school and taught for two and a half years. I was teaching along with some of the same people who fought to keep me labeled "retarded".

Then I spent the next two years coaching at Lincoln University as an assistant football coach and director of the athletic dormitory.

From there, I returned to Denmark to coach professional basketball and learn Danish. The Chernobyl nuclear disaster brought me back home.

I have since been a teacher at Residential Rehabilitation Centers on Cape Cod. Here I'm giving love and concern to people I know a great deal about. It is very strange for me to be teaching mentally retarded people. I can't help but reflect back to my years as a mentally retarded person, and how things could have turned out if I were still living in foster care homes. But that was then, and this is now.

To Kathy, Joan and Paul, I say "Thank You!"

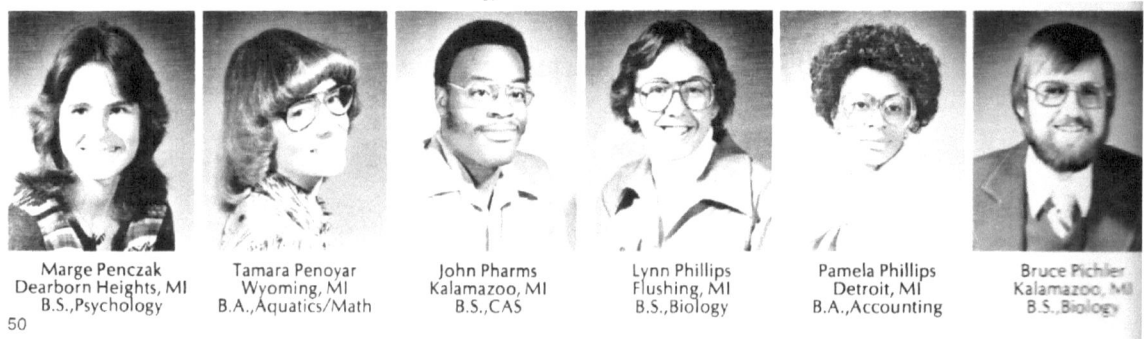

Marge Penczak
Dearborn Heights, MI
B.S.,Psychology
50

Tamara Penoyar
Wyoming, MI
B.A.,Aquatics/Math

John Pharms
Kalamazoo, MI
B.S.,CAS

Lynn Phillips
Flushing, MI
B.S.,Biology

Pamela Phillips
Detroit, MI
B.A.,Accounting

Bruce Pichler
Kalamazoo, MI
B.S.,Biology

This is me graduating from Western Michigan University in June of 1977.
(Third from the left)

Bibliography

Coldwater, "The Daily Reporter", 1963

Fort Custer, "As You Were", 1985

"Gazette", Kalamazoo, 1986

Medical Report, 1989

Psychological Report, 1988

2014

Where Am I Now

As I look back on such a difficult upbringing, I'm reminded of two films that have nailed me on target. The first film, "One Flew over the Cuckoo's Nest" with Jack Nicholson, reminded me of my institutional Years in the old Fort Custer State Home in Battle Creek, Michigan and the former Coldwater State Home in Coldwater, Michigan. There were homes for the mentally and physically retarded. I was born at eight months and weighed three pounds. I became a ward of the State of Michigan at ten months and stayed that way until I was 19.

If you ever saw that film, you will be astonished that I ever made it out of there alive! The book that you're reading doesn't come close to depicting all the events that I grew up experiencing. Many beatings, viewing my first dead body (at the age of eight), severe beatings on my genitals and much more harrowing experiences too gruesome to mention.

The second film is "Prozac Nation" with Christina Ricci. As I'm penning these last thoughts, I am watching "Proac Nation" for only the second time! I just can't watch it. I've been on Prozac for a number of years. Suicide thoughts have plagued me since I walked between a school bus and city bus walking home as a 9th grader. My doctor changed my medication to where I went from thinking of suicide ten times a day to its non-existence today. I tell my friends that if you want to know who I am, watch this film. It chronicles my life from foster care, special education classes, being teased un mercifully because of my eye were crossed, and a severe stutter that made it very difficult for anyone to understand what I was saying to a retired teacher.

I won a first place ribbon in a riding competition. Won a part on the old *Unsolved Mysteries* television show while living on Cape Cod, made a small movie in Europe for French children's Television Show, and taught in Mallorca, Spain and Denmark while doing summer work in Amsterdam.

Though I've never been married with no children of my own, I do count thousands of kids I've been blessed to know. Though marriage was never in my plans I have been intimate with a very lovely lady name Sherry for nearly 13 years.

I hope you're touched by this story, and that you will share it with others less fortunate as I was.

I hope this book touches just one kid who will one day grow up to be nominated for Citizen of the Year as I was in 2003 in my home town of Jackson, Michigan.

Though these three women are now deceased, I want to Thank Nora Clardy, Peg Doyle and Cleo Mae Dungy (Tony Dungy's mother) for getting me out of special education class as a 10th grader and Herb Furnace for fighting hard to get me into Western Michigan University.

The Untold Yet Remarkable Story of a Very Determined Little Boy Named Johnnie

About John Pharms

Refusing to accept derogatory titles attached to him by society and determined to make it in an often cruel and unfriendly world, John Pharms, a ward of the courts of the State of Michigan at the age of ten months, stands today as testimony to the virtue of self-determination.

The 6'3" pound former athlete, who today teaches G.E.D. classes for the Michigan Department of Corrections has come a long way from that day, over fifty year ago, when he and his twin brother Jimmy were mad permanent custody as wards of the State of Michigan from their natural parents. John Pharms spent many years being reared in State Institution, Foster Care Homes, Boarding Homes and, for a short stint, with their Uncle Frank and Aunt Billy in Grand Rapids, Michigan. Spending years with the mentally and physically challenged children was an unpromising start to life, one that might have depressed and finished many others, but not John Pharms.

After receiving his discharge papers from the State of Michigan and upon receiving his high school diploma form Jackson High School, John Pharms entered Western Michigan University, where he received a scholarship, alone, confused and wondering if he had made a mistake. Large lecture halls, college math, introduction to drugs and alcohol was all to consuming for one just removed from special education classes, but John Pharms went on to concurred those obstacles and graduated after completing his student teaching on an island called Mallorca, Spain.

John Pharms was assisting Western Michigan's Track Program when he head men's track coach, Jack Shaw, shared with him that his formed high school track coach, Charlie Janke, was looking for an assistant to help him with the track program there at Jackson High School. Without hesitating, John Pharms saw this opportunity as a way to return to his alma mater as a teacher and coach!

John Pharms returned to his alma mater where he taught and coached athletics along with some of the same educators who refused to acknowledge that he should never have been labeled a special education student in the first place. After nearly three years at his alma mater, John pharms decided to take his talents to the University Level. Tony Dungy, head football coach for the Indianapolis Colt Football Team, referred John Pharms (Pharms and Dungy were from the same city of Jackson, Michigan where they competed in sports against each other) to Lincoln University in Jefferson City, Missouri where Pharms would be Dorm Director for the athlete's dormitory, equipment manager, assistant football coach and professor through Lincoln where he taught English at the local Prison. It was also there that Pharms met and became acquainted with the late Archie Moore (former light heavyweight boxing champion) through his son Hardy who resided in the Tiger Football Team. Hardy would later pass away from cancer.

After another two-year stint at Lincoln, Pharms returned back to Mallorca, Spain where he had done his student teaching before graduating from Western Michigan. After two years there where Pharms was the house father for the boys dormitory, athletic director, theater director, coached the boys and girls athletic teams, Pharms decided that it was time to accept another offer and returned to Arhus, Denmark where he was a summer exchange student while also attending Western Michigan.

John Pharms accepted to coach the Division 1 Basketball Team after visiting his host family (from his college days) over the Christmas Holidays. After coaching and teaching in the Danish School System, Pharms decided that it was time to come home. After turning down an offer to play and coach basketball in Poland, Pharms returned to Jackson, Michigan where, after only a six-month stay, decided to follow a high school classmate to Raleigh, North Carolina. John Pharms had a Job as a manager of a dry cleaning establishment in a small town call Ajax, North Carolina. John Pharms decided, after nearly six months living in North Carolina, decided to pay a visit to a friend from Denmark.

John Pharms made his way to the home of lone time friend Steve Oliver on Cape Cod, planning only on a two-week visit, but after nearly five years (remember the three hour tour from the Gillian's Island Television Program?) Pharms decided again that it was time to return home! It was back to Jackson, Michigan where Pharms would receive his Master's Degree from Spring Arbor University, retire as a full-time teacher for the Michigan Department of Corrections and receive many accolades one being nominated for "Citizen of the Year" for his work with Jackson County's Youth.

Though John Pharms has never been married and has no children of his own, many present and former athletes/students look upon John Pharms has a role model and mentor, John Pharms has found time to give back to society many times over.

To order books written by John Pharms please Google Johnnie Pharms LULU. For speaking engagements you may contact John Pharms at johnpharms@gmail.com.